"This is a great story of an adventurous and wide-ranging doctor dedicated to bringing the human into medicine. Having felt the whip of money and 'administrators,' in both large institutions and small hospitals, she and Simon Talbot moved away from calling doctors' difficulties 'burnout' — thus blaming doctors — to 'moral injury' — like soldiers floundering under unjust orders. A brilliant, expansive book."
— Samuel Shem, MD, DPhil, Professor in Medicine at NYU Medical School, author of *The House of God* and *Man's 4th Best Hospital*

"A manifesto for our times! Wendy Dean diagnoses the dangerous state of our healthcare system, illustrating the thumbscrews applied to medical professionals by their corporate overlords. By making it impossible to do the right thing for patients, the profit-hungry system casually gouges the moral fiber of healthcare workers, threatening patient safety. Luckily, Dean lays out a path forward. Required reading for all stakeholders in healthcare."
— Danielle Ofri, MD, PhD, author of *When We Do Harm: A Doctor Confronts Medical Error*

"Wendy Dean offers a stunning portrayal of the corrosive effects of valuing profits over people. Medicine is sick and the situation more dire than most realize, but Dean's examples of visionary leadership inspire hope for a healthier future. Written by *the* expert on moral injury in medicine, this book is a critical read for all in healthcare.»
— Lydia Dugdale, MD, author of *The Lost Art of Dying: Reviving Forgotten Wisdom*, Director of the Center for Clinical Medical Ethics at Columbia University

"All good physicians embrace their role as 'Chief Story Teller,' explaining to patients and their families the meaning of symptoms, diagnostic tests and proposed treatments. Wendy Dean weaves together the stories of 13 healthcare clinicians who have grappled with moral injury resulting from the system in which they are forced to work, and also offers solutions. A brilliantly conceived and executed masterpiece."

— Thom Mayer, MD, Medical Director
of the NFL Players Association

"I was viscerally moved by this book. Although written by and about the challenges facing physicians in the civilian healthcare system, I shared many similarly exasperating experiences during my military medical career. Wendy Dean opens the door for the layman to see how physically taxing and mentally draining the practice of medicine can be, while allowing physician readers to recognize themselves in the scenarios she depicts. Regardless of where you stand, you need to read this book. Trust me. I'm a doctor."

— Joseph Caravalho, Jr., MD, Major General,
US Army (Retired), President and CEO of
the Henry M. Jackson Foundation for the
Advancement of Military Medicine

IF I BETRAY
THESE WORDS

Moral Injury in Medicine and Why
It's So Hard for Clinicians to Put Patients First

WENDY DEAN, M.D.
with
SIMON TALBOT, M.D.

STEERFORTH PRESS
LEBANON, NEW HAMPSHIRE

For information about permission to reproduce
selections from this book, write to:
Steerforth Press L.L.C., 31 Hanover Street, Suite 1
Lebanon, New Hampshire 03766

Cataloging-in-Publication Data is available from the Library of Congress

ISBN 978-1-58642-354-4

Printed in the United States of America

For patients and clinicians, who all deserve better.

For Austin and Caleb, who are why I love and fight so fiercely.

And for Shervin, who has always said I should write a book.
I used to think he loved me.

Contents

Author's Note

The deadline for choosing a title for this book arrived unexpectedly as I was deep into writing chapter 6, which is about a doctor who takes his own life. In a flurry of communications with the publisher and editor that grew more frantic by the hour, we tried to distill the essence of the work to a word or two. The collected stories deserved exactly the right title, but despair about a flurry of imperfect ideas melded with the grief I was feeling about the character in chapter 6, and I was lost.

As I often do when stuck in a morass, I paused and returned to the source document, so to speak — to the oath we take as physicians, in its many forms. This oath represents what each of us believes is our duty to society in joining this profession and embarking on a lifetime of tending to strangers in their moments of greatest vulnerability and need. It is the commitment that calls us to be our best selves.

I read the Declaration of Geneva of the World Medical Association, the Oath of the Healer, the American Medical Association Code of Medical Ethics, the Osteopathic Oath, the Maimonides Prayer, and many versions of the Hippocratic Oath. Similar themes ran through them all: gratitude toward teachers, a commitment to lifelong learning, an obligation to nurture the next generation, selflessness, one's duty to patients above all else, honesty, humility, confidentiality, love. But when I discovered a 2010 translation of the Hippocratic Oath by Amelia Arenas, published in Boston University's journal *Arion*, I found the title.

This version of the oath echoes the themes of all the rest, but the last lines took my breath away (emphasis added):

I pray that the attention I give to those who put themselves in my hands be rewarded with happiness. And in honor of the knowledge I've received from my teachers, I swear to care for anyone who suffers, prince or slave.

If I ever break this oath, let my gods take away my knowledge of this art and my own health.

Here speaks a citizen, a servant of people. *May I be destroyed if I betray these words.*

The covenant we make is not simply about how we will do a job, it is also about who we will be when we don the mantel of "physician." It prescribes our conduct, calibrates our moral compass, and entwines both with our identity. Betraying these words, then, forsakes our identity, which can unmoor us and threaten our dissolution.

In standing up to moral injury and fighting for our oaths, we are fighting for our patients as if our lives depend on it. Because, figuratively, and too often literally, they do.

I am humbled by and grateful to all the medical professionals who have spoken up against their destruction, and to those who find the courage to do so in the future.

What Beer and Modern Healthcare Have in Common

Dr. Mike Hilden answered the knock on his front door in the fall of 2012 to find two Federal Bureau of Investigation (FBI) agents waiting to speak with him. The FBI hadn't come to Carlisle, a quiet college town of twenty thousand people in central Pennsylvania, for drug dealers or old-school racketeers. They were talking to doctors, nurses, and administrators at the local hospital, tipped off by whistleblowers who leveled fraud allegations at Health Management Associates (HMA), the fourth-largest hospital corporation in the United States, and the owner of Carlisle Regional Medical Center.

Dr. Hilden had been a hospitalist at Carlisle Regional for more than a decade, since before the board of the nonprofit community hospital sold out to HMA. Now it was one of seventy-one hospitals in a nationwide for-profit enterprise that was being accused of coercing physicians to forsake their medical judgment — to hospitalize patients who didn't meet insurance criteria, to order more tests than their conditions required, and to keep them in the hospital longer than necessary — to increase profits.

Carlisle, established by Scots Irish in the mid-eighteenth century, had an early history fraught with conflict. The Carlisle Barracks, now home to the United States Army War College, served as supply headquarters in the Revolutionary War. George Washington reviewed troops there before sending them west to put down the Whiskey Rebellion, and downtown buildings still bear the scars of a three-day occupation by Robert E. Lee during the Civil War. But since stopping the northward advance of the Confederate army, the town had been a quiet place. Unfortunately, though the community didn't know it yet, the fight in healthcare over profits, patients, and physician autonomy, waged by ever-larger corporations, was coming to them.

A key figure in the FBI investigation was someone few people in Carlisle had ever heard of: HMA board chairman William Schoen. Just a few months earlier, at the company's annual shareholders' meeting at a Ritz-Carlton resort in Naples, Florida, Schoen defended himself against a few shareholders agitating for his ouster. The disgruntled shareholders claimed that HMA failed to hold its executives to the same standards as competing corporations and that its insufficient attention to compliance with federal regulations put the corporation at risk.

Under Schoen, HMA's only criterion for executive bonuses was a single financial measure: EBITDA (earnings before interest, taxes, depreciation, and amortization), a measure that isn't one of the generally accepted accounting principles used by publicly traded companies in financial statements. Moreover, most large, publicly traded healthcare corporations also included at least one quality indicator, such as readmission rates, hospital-acquired infections, or patient satisfaction, in bonus calculations.[1] Charlie Munger, vice president of Warren Buffett's Berkshire Hathaway, in his 2020 address to the *Daily Journal* shareholders meeting, referred to EBITDA as "bullshit earnings," a measure so manipulable it deserves little credence.[2] Shareholders were concerned that HMA executives were manipulating the numbers to line their own pockets rather than creating real value for investors, while a weak board, whose members were handpicked by Schoen and secure in their tenure, was doing nothing about it.

During his time as chief executive officer and board chairman, Schoen had grown the organization from a small regional player to a Fortune 500 company with national reach and billions in revenue. His responsibility was to his shareholders, not to clinicians, and not to patients, who were both free to go elsewhere if they didn't like the conditions at his hospitals. Schoen believed that his compensation, and that of his senior team, was hardly out of line with their success, or with their peers in the industry.

At the meeting, HMA's vice president of financial relations at the time, John Merriwether, denied the critics' contentions: "To imply that we don't take quality as seriously as we should, that's not fair. If you don't provide good quality care, you won't have good financial performance."[3] But HMA specifically targeted markets where it knew there was little or no competition, so patients at HMA hospitals could not vote with their feet or their healthcare dollars. The Center for American Progress found that rural emergency rooms in hospitals like those HMA acquired were, on average, twenty-two miles from the next nearest emergency room,[4] a distance that could mean the difference between life and death.

Ultimately, the shareholders weren't swayed by the critics. Schoen, the board, and the compensation structure all remained unchanged. But the Health Care Fraud Prevention and Enforcement Action Team, a joint effort by the US Department of Justice and the US secretary of health and human services, was just getting started with HMA. Between 2009 and 2011, whistleblowers filed eight lawsuits against the corporation, alleging fraud. Agents from the FBI and Department of Justice spent two years talking with hundreds of employees across at least eight states, and by the time the investigation was over, HMA agreed to pay a $260 million settlement for forcing doctors, under threat of losing their jobs, to provide unnecessary care against their best judgment and training. Dr. Hilden was vindicated, but he and his partners, like so many other physicians in the grip of increasingly corporatized healthcare, were looking for new jobs — ones where they could practice medicine as they had been trained to do, not as corporate growth plans told them they must.

William Schoen grew up during the Great Depression in Arcadia, Florida. Even as a child, he was resourceful: selling flower seeds at eight years old; hawking newspapers at the racetrack at thirteen; and

dropping out of high school to start a scrap metal business. During the
Korean War, he enlisted in the marines. Unhappy serving on the front
lines, he vowed to finish his education when he got home. He eventually earned a master's degree in business administration, studying
lean management principles and how economies of scale benefit the
bottom line, and upon graduation went straight into the turbulent,
low-margin world of glassmaking as a marketing manager for Anchor
Hocking.[5] In less than a decade, he became president and CEO of
Pierce Glass, where his ambition caught the eye of Robert Lear, CEO
of the holding company that owned Pierce.[6] When family-run brewer
F&M Schaefer Corporation recruited Lear to turn around their falter-
ing beer business in 1972, Lear jumped at the chance but knew he
couldn't do it alone. He started planning how to bring Schoen on at
Schaefer.

Businesses usually succeed in one of three ways: through better quality, lower cost, or less competition. Until the mid-twentieth century,
most beer was locally brewed, and companies balanced quality and
cost to appeal to local tastes. By the 1960s, however, companies like
Anheuser-Busch, Schlitz, Pabst, and Miller had built industrial breweries, churning out beer at one-quarter the cost of local breweries, in
strategic locations along the new interstate highway system, which
enabled them to ship their cheap, bland brew around the country.[7]

Brothers Frederick and Maximilian Schaefer, immigrants from
Germany, founded F&M Schaefer Brewing in New York City in 1846.
The company survived the Civil War, Prohibition, and the privations
of two world wars, but by the late 1960s, it was struggling. An attempt
to expand Schaefer's regional market into Ohio had failed. Brewing
was consolidating, with companies leveraging economies of scale
to compete on cost. Schaefer's breweries in Albany, Brooklyn, and
Baltimore were aging and inefficient. To compete with the big brands,
then CEO Rudolph Schaefer II, grandson of Maximilian, decided
to build a new brewery. To fund the project, he needed cash,[8] so in
1968 he took the company public, raising $106 million in capital. In

taking the company public, F&M Schaefer Brewing was split into two business entities: F&M Schaefer Corporation, the parent holding company, and Schaefer Brewing Company, the production subsidiary. Schaefer immediately spent $60 million building a modern brewery near major transportation hubs in Fogelsville, Pennsylvania, just outside the former steel powerhouse of Allentown, where land was cheap and labor was plentiful, with so many steel workers recently laid off.

During the four years of construction, from 1968 to 1972, the company continued to lose market share to the national brands.[9] When the new brewery finally started sending out beer, customers complained they could taste a difference. Sales flagged and debts mounted. Something had to change.

Enter Robert Lear. Just a year after he was brought in, Lear lured Schoen away from Pierce Glass to oversee the production subsidiary, Schaefer Brewing, displacing Rudie Schaefer III. Rudie had been with the company for sixteen years, working his way up the ranks as an expert in production, and was being groomed to take over from his father.[10] But Lear and Schoen dismissed Rudie's expertise. Their goal wasn't quality, it was survival as a profitable company. Lear was confident that Schoen's "record of making his own way, overcoming problems, and meeting formidable challenges" would make up for his lack of experience in the beer industry.[11] But Rudie couldn't bear to watch his family name associated with a shoddy product. In 1976, after three years of working with men who didn't value his expertise, Rudie told his father the work was "untenable" and left. The younger Schaefer never returned to brewing.[12]

When the Fogelsville brewery opened in 1972, Rudie Schaefer had closed the Albany facility, and three hundred people lost their jobs. Still plagued by falling market share in 1976, Schoen needed to cut expenses further. He again increased production in Fogelsville, then shuttered the Brooklyn plant, putting another 850 employees on the street.

Schaefer had tried competing first with better quality, then with lower cost, both unsuccessfully. So Schoen looked to the third strategy: less competition. With the bigger brands dominating most of the mainland US market, he set his sights on the island of Puerto Rico, where beer consumption per capita had doubled in the 1960s, but competition from local breweries was limited. By 1977, Schaefer held 70 percent of the beer market in Puerto Rico, and its Baltimore brewery was shipping 1.3 million barrels of beer to the island every year, amounting to a third of Schaefer's entire business.[13]

Then in 1978, after years of rumors it would happen, legislators in Puerto Rico imposed a five-cent-per-can excise tax on imports from large breweries, which undercut Schaefer's price advantage in that market. A third of Schaefer's business evaporated overnight, and Schoen needed to cut overhead sharply, so he closed the Baltimore brewery and put three hundred more workers on the street.[14] Spooked, and out of ideas for how to recover, Schoen started eyeing the exits.

On Thursday, May 14, 1981, after barely eight years at the company, Schoen completed the sale of Schaefer to Stroh Brewing, which wanted the Fogelsville brewery to expand production of its own beer. He walked away with, as the *Tampa Bay Times* put it, "a pile of money" from his time as CEO, but the deal he struck was less a windfall for shareholders than a way to save face and avoid bankruptcy. In less than a decade, William Schoen, who knew nothing about the beer industry, took a family business that had been around for a century and a half and sold it for parts. Schaefer beer was no more.

Schoen had been semi-retired and working as a consultant for less than two years when twenty-eight-year-old Kent Dauten asked him to join the board of directors of Naples, Florida–based HMA, which at the time owned twelve hospitals. Dauten had joined First Chicago Venture Capital in Chicago two years earlier, after graduating from Harvard with an MBA, and HMA was his first investment for the firm. He'd gambled on the founder, Joseph Greene, who had deep experience in healthcare, but his business principles were unorthodox, and HMA had been losing money on its urban hospitals. Dauten had heard rumors about a guy in Naples who managed a tough turn-around in a low-margin industry and made a king's ransom in the process. How different could brewing be from healthcare? Balance sheets were balance sheets.

Greene, formerly the president of hospital operations at Humana, founded HMA in 1977; he ran the company as a family business, with his brother and son in leadership roles. An evangelical Christian, he applied biblical principles to his business practices, going so far as to develop a "Ministry Plan" for how the corporation would serve not only its patients but also its employees and its vendors.[15] For exam-ple, he insisted that every bill be paid within twenty-four hours, to avoid using money owed to someone else — "borrowing from Peter to pay Paul." More traditional accounting practices delayed payment until nearly the due date to let the capital work by accruing interest.[16] Greene's practices cut into profit margins and frustrated shareholders, like Dauten's investment bank, who started agitating for change.

Within months of Schoen joining the board in 1983, his fellow board members elected him president and chief operating officer of the company. He brought in $7 million in outside investments to shore up the company's financial position, and in 1985, the board elevated him to co-CEO with Greene. Fed up with constant conflict with Schoen, Greene stepped down just months later.[17] Once again, someone with deep industry expertise was out of the picture in one of Schoen's ventures, and he had free rein to run a company in a sector he knew nothing about.

Schoen even admitted as much. "I came from the beer business with no preconceived idea other than that monopoly was good."[18] His first move as CEO was to sell off ten of the company's twelve hospi-tals, mostly in competitive urban markets. Those hospitals may have aligned with Joseph Greene's Christian intent to help the needy, but they had a poor payer mix (few patients with private insurance, too many uninsured) and were dragging HMA's balance sheet into the red. They had to go.

Then he started rebuilding, buying up ailing community hospitals in rural areas where population growth guaranteed strong demand and a lack of competition meant HMA would own the market. These small hospitals typically operated at low margins, if they made any profit; after all, they existed to serve their communities. But Schoen was confident that he could turn them into moneymakers for HMA. The *Tampa Bay Times* described the HMA formula as "simple, but capital-intensive."

> Improve patient-grabbing basics such as obstetrics and the emergency room. Add more sophisticated services to keep residents from taking their business to the nearest big city. And recruit more specialists and sub-specialists.
>
> At the same time, HMA squeezes cost out of its hospitals by volume purchasing and by hooking up hospitals to a computerized information system that tracks everything from lab use to patient billing. HMA also cuts labor costs by relying heavily on flextime. In other words, its hospitals send nurses home when the patient count is low and load them up with overtime during peak winter months.[19]

At the start of Schoen's tenure, most healthcare executives were nervous about how impending changes to Medicare reimbursement would affect profitability. Instead of paying hospitals according to the care they rendered, which can encourage overtreatment, Medicare would soon begin reimbursing at a fixed rate according to the patient's diagnosis, known as diagnosis-related group payments. More-experienced healthcare executives knew that these fixed rates were calculated based on careful estimates of what it cost hospitals to treat various conditions, but Schoen was unfazed. Provided that HMA cut costs below the Medicare rate, kept more of its beds full, or some combination of the two, Schoen saw fixed prices as guaranteed profit.[20] He controlled large parts of each hospital's overhead with group purchasing; installed software to direct and monitor patient care; established goals for admissions, testing, and revenue; then told local hospital leadership they'd lose their jobs if they didn't keep up.

Meanwhile, HMA invested in superficial improvements, like updating lobbies and offering senior citizen discounts in the cafeteria, designed to increase patient satisfaction. As Andrea Robbins wrote in *The Atlantic* in 2015: "Many hospitals seem to be highly focused on pixie-dusted sleight of hand because they believe they can trick patients into thinking they got better care . . . the smoke and mirrors serve to distract from the real problem."[21] By 2012, HMA had acquired seventy-one hospitals in fourteen states and was one of the most profitable healthcare companies in the country.

Schoen's relentless focus on profit also had consequences for doctors at HMA hospitals. HMA pressured all its physicians to increase revenue, but the problem was particularly acute in emergency rooms. Shifts previously staffed by two physicians were now covered by just one. When a patient entered an emergency room at an HMA hospital, nurses entered their information into the computer, which automatically ordered extensive batteries of tests, called protocols, under the emergency physician's name, before the physician had even seen the patient. Physicians are taught that all testing should occur in a stepwise fashion, based on a differential diagnosis of the most likely conditions. Testing confirms or refutes that differential; it doesn't substitute for it. Besides the risk of harm inherent in any test — from benign anxiety to permanent impairment — overtesting inflicts financial harm from excessive copays. Many of the tests automatically ordered in HMA emergency rooms were unnecessary once the physician saw the patient, but it was too late to stop them. The company also set targets for hospital admissions and strong-armed doctors to meet them.

If doctors at HMA hospitals had complained — to an administrator, supervisor, or colleague — about the difficulty of caring for patients under such conditions, they might have been dismissed as burned out. In other words, they just didn't have what it took to hack this job.

But the deep distress these doctors felt was something that went beyond burnout. Doctors were being pressured to practice in ways that went against their conscience and their training, and patient care was suffering. If they spoke up about what was happening, they might lose their jobs. Schoen fired the CEO of one local hospital in 2009 for telling his physicians to "do what you think is best for the patient," rather than meeting the targets HMA set.[22] And if they lost their jobs, where else in their rural communities could they find work without uprooting their families?

Sadly, doctors were right to worry about patient harm. Understaffing likely contributed to at least two deaths in Mike Hilden's hospital in Pennsylvania in 2011.[23] From 2009 through 2011, former HMA staff across the country, including physicians, administrators, and executives, filed eight separate whistleblower lawsuits alleging years of Medicare fraud throughout the HMA healthcare system. In December 2013, the Department of Justice had sufficient evidence to join the suits and moved them to Washington, DC, for litigation. The FBI agents who showed up on Mike Hilden's doorstep were part of the investigation, as were US attorneys in seven states, the Health and Human Services Office of the Inspector General, and the Defense Health Agency Program Integrity.[24] In July 2013, the CEO of HMA, Gary Newsome, abruptly resigned.

In mid-August 2013, Glenview Capital Management, a $6 billion hedge fund in New York City, initiated the process to oust the board. Glenview argued that HMA was not maximizing shareholder value, and the board was not taking sufficient corrective action. The majority of shareholders agreed.[25] William Schoen was out, along with the rest of the board.

Just before his ouster, Schoen negotiated a $7.6 billion buyout of HMA by Community Health Systems, which was finalized in 2014,[26] in which he walked away with a severance deal of $1 million per year, use of a private jet, and a treasure chest of tens of millions in stock options amassed during his thirty-year career.[27] After the merger, Wayne Smith, the new chairman and CEO, said, "We look forward to effectively integrating this acquisition and generating significant value for our shareholders."[28]

William Schoen seems like a remarkable character, worthy of a book of his own. But the sobering fact is that he was in the vanguard of thousands of executives who moved into healthcare as other sectors consolidated and offshored. Schoen's ilk extracted massive profits for themselves and their associates by manipulating the mission of health-care, exploiting the altruism of their workforce, and taking advantage of patients at their most defenseless and vulnerable time.

I grew up in western Massachusetts, where I spent my childhood on the go — climbing trees, playing pickup sports, riding horses, and mucking stalls to pay for lessons. My father was a self-employed trav-eling salesman, peddling fasteners and cable to manufacturers like General Electric, Sikorsky, and Raytheon. My mother was his secre-tary and bookkeeper, as her mother had been for her father's plumb-ing business. Though I did clerical and cleaning tasks for the business, my father made it clear from the very beginning that I had no future there; my brother, six years older, was being groomed to take over. Shut out of the family business, I declared at nine years old I would be a doctor, much to my parents' disbelief.

In high school, I shadowed a local pediatrician and volunteered at the community hospital; in college, I discovered the *Journal of Bone and Joint Surgery* and read every issue cover-to-cover. Drawn to the physics of orthopedics and the immediate gratification of "cutting to cure," I shadowed a local orthopedic surgeon the summer after my freshman year. By the time I graduated from medical school at the University of Massachusetts in 1991, my goal had shifted to plastic surgery, and I began a five-year general surgery residency at Dartmouth Hitchcock Medical Center in Hanover, New Hampshire, to qualify for a three-year plastic surgery fellowship. Three years in, I realized that no matter how much I loved it, or how good I was at it, surgery was not right for me. Surgeons excel through repetition, honing their craft by doing the same procedures time after time, whereas I thrive on novelty. More than that, when I realized the reconstructive practice I'd planned was so poorly reimbursed that breast augmentation, tummy tucks, and face-lifts would need to subsidize it, I reconsidered. I left for work in rural emergency rooms to catch my breath, pay my bills, and decide what was next, including whether I could even stay in medicine.

The one thing I was absolutely sure about that year was the man I first met in the summer of 1993 when he started his neurosurgery internship. Initially skeptical that anyone could be as smart, competent, and kind as my neurosurgery friends said this guy was, when we started dating in the early winter, I soon realized that Shervin was all they promised, and more. After a whirlwind courtship, he proposed just weeks before I resigned my residency, and we married the next fall.

Emergency medicine offered the variety I craved — earaches, intentional poisoning, terrible car wrecks, chain-saw accidents, self-castration, falls, strokes, heart attacks, and plenty of animal bites. By the end of my first year, I realized two things: I still wanted to be a doctor, and my satisfaction came from forming relationships with patients, knowing who they were, not just how they were suffering, and bearing witness to the course of their illness. The emergency room was not a place for that.

The psychiatry patients who presented in crisis drew me. The relationship with the patient was the primary tool for both diagnosis and treatment, and the biological underpinnings of the disorders were just beginning to emerge. The field would evolve rapidly, probably for my whole career, which would keep me engaged. Finally, an outpatient psychiatry practice does not require any special equipment, facilities, or assistants. If I couldn't find a job that suited me, I could rent an office, hang out my shingle, and practice exactly as I was trained to do.

In the fall of 1996, I returned to residency at Dartmouth, this time in psychiatry. I chose Dartmouth, in part, for its strong reputation of training excellent psychotherapists. In the 1990s, managed care, which was wreaking havoc in general medicine, was particularly destructive to mental health care, slashing reimbursement by 54 percent as opposed to the 11.5 percent cut to general medical services.[29] Revenue in Dartmouth's psychiatry program faced a crisis because, like all other psychiatry programs, revenue had fallen precipitously, but the hospital, strained by cuts across the board, had decreed that every department had to at least cover its costs.

In response, the department hired Dr. Leighton Huey as vice chair to turn the department around the year before I arrived. Huey had a reputation for being unapologetic about pursuing his vision of the future: psychiatrists with "a sense of fiscal realities and . . . the implications of health care reform and managed care."[30] Psychiatrists should manage medication (the biology) and leave therapy (the psychosocial aspects of treatment) to other clinicians. He was also an advocate of hustle culture. If we wanted to gain the respect of surgeons, he said, we had to work as hard as they did.

The pace of my psychiatry residency turned out to be very similar to my surgical residency, although the call nights were fewer and easier. By the time I was in my next-to-last year, I ran from a morning of caring for psychiatry inpatients and supervising junior residents to a medication management clinic with as many as twenty outpatients in the afternoon. Most days I returned to the hospital — a quarter mile away — multiple times to do psychiatric assessments of patients admitted for medical or surgical conditions. Training in psychotherapy was sharply curtailed, but I refused to give up on what I viewed as an essential part of training, so I added extra hours every week to learn psychotherapy from clinicians in private practice in the community.

Six months before I finished residency, and shortly after giving birth to my first child, I started looking for employment at a large hospital that offered opportunities for career advancement. I would be supporting our family while Shervin, who had recently resigned his neurosurgery residency, stayed home and cared for our son. After interviewing for several jobs, I was offered the position of director of the Emergency Psychiatry Service at Rhode Island Hospital, part of Lifespan, the state's first health system, established in 1994. Before accepting, I did my due diligence and confirmed the position was as advertised, so we moved to Providence.

But as many of my friends found in their first jobs, the position was not what I expected. The service was under-resourced — just me, a very competent nurse practitioner, and an administrative assistant unqualified to help with insurance prior authorizations, the most time-intensive part of my job. For every thirty minutes I spent with a patient, I spent ninety minutes or more trying to convince insurance companies to pay for a hospital admission my training and expertise deemed necessary, and another hour calling hospital after hospital looking for one that would accept the admission. The reimbursement cuts in mental health care over the previous decade had hit Rhode Island as hard as everywhere else, and competition among organizations to bring in well-insured patients, while avoiding the under-insured, was cutthroat. The pressure to avoid admitting uninsured patients, which would have meant a financial loss for the hospital, sometimes bordered on unethical to me, though my bosses dismissed my concerns. When I learned, after several months, that there was no opportunity for advancement because of a quirk in how they'd funded the position, I was done.

As the sole earner for my young family paying off two sets of student loans, I was in no position to be an activist. But I was not willing to compromise my ethics or the standard of care I had been trained to provide. Shervin supported my objection, even if it meant making personal sacrifices to do it. After less than a year in that job

I decided that navigating the politics and financial imperatives of a big hospital that were tangled in the politics of a notoriously corrupt city, all of which interfered with my ability to care for patients, was not for me.

Shervin and I decided to move back to Hanover, New Hampshire. He would return to a radiology residency at Dartmouth the following year, and the area had enough demand to keep another private-practice psychiatrist busy. The community highly valued mental health care and was wealthy enough that patients could afford the higher costs of seeing clinicians outside their insurance network. I still had enough connections with colleagues in the area that my practice filled quickly. The trade-off for autonomy and latitude, though, was shouldering all the financial risk and responsibility of the practice, while being on call for my patients every day, all year long. But the freedom to practice with integrity was a profound relief. For the four years of Shervin's residency, my practice supported our family.

In 2006, Shervin finished his training and we moved to Carlisle, Pennsylvania, for his first job as a radiologist. I opened another solo practice but soon learned that insurance plans were not as generous, the area was less affluent, and patients were more reluctant to seek out-of-network care. Insurance paid one rate for psychotherapy, whether a social worker, psychologist, or psychiatrist provided it. But my malpractice costs were ten times higher because I could be held responsible for other clinicians' care.[31] If I agreed to take insurance and accept their payment for psychotherapy, I would struggle to keep the practice viable. The best way to ensure a viable practice was to give up doing psychotherapy, accept insurance, and only see patients for medication management. Stubbornly hoping to create the niche I'd found in New Hampshire, I tried to do psychotherapy half the time and medication management the other half, but after five years of struggling, I closed the practice. I still loved the work I did with patients, but I couldn't justify the liability while only breaking even, and I couldn't make more money without compromising my care.

When I closed my practice in 2011, I took a job with the US Army, managing research funding for regenerative medicine and hand and face transplants. As part of our oversight, my office held monthly conference calls with physicians in various specialties at many different healthcare systems across the country. I also saw many of them several times each year at conferences. These colleagues were at the top of their fields, doctors deeply committed to the practice of medicine and who genuinely enjoyed caring for patients. But in unguarded moments, over dinner or drinks, many confessed to being increasingly unhappy in their jobs. They signed up for hard work and long hours, but lately the pace had accelerated dramatically: They were seeing more patients, in less time, with fewer support staff, and they were required to use technology that interfered with rather than facilitated care. In our conversations, many of these doctors were speaking frankly about their frustrations for the first time.

For years, hospitals had been surveying their staff about their levels of fatigue, frustration, or disengagement, using tools like the Maslach Burnout Inventory. The consistency of findings across disparate organizations led to a 2018 report by Harvard University and the Massachusetts Medical Society, which declared physician burnout a "public health crisis."[32] Ostensibly, the goal of the inventory was to better understand the phenomenon of workplace distress; in practice, it was often used to identify outliers with high scores — in the burnout range — and manage the risk they represented to the organization, since burnout is associated with lower quality of care and lower productivity.[33] Employers encouraged these physicians to seek out programs — meditation, mindfulness, yoga, or others — that would help them build resilience and learn to take better care of themselves, though there was no data proving these programs were effective at relieving the distress.[34] If doctors didn't follow recommendations, they could be labeled as difficult or impaired (a term usually reserved for those with substance use disorders) by their burnout, which could put their medical license in jeopardy.[35]

While the doctors I spoke to were admittedly exhausted, they were adamant that their personal mental health was not the issue. Something had gone terribly wrong with our healthcare system, and it was causing them profound distress. If it wasn't burnout, though, what was it?

The question nagged at me for months until one spring day in 2016, I was weeding the garden when I heard a guest on public radio describe how service members returning from Iraq and Afghanistan were not responding to PTSD treatments known to be effective. Through deeper interviews and consulting research on Vietnam veterans, the researcher realized these veterans were not experiencing anxiety and avoidance caused by fear but rather shame and guilt associated with perceived immoral conduct. To help them, clinicians needed a better description of the nature of the traumatic experience that was causing the veterans' distress. What they came up with was moral injury: "perpetrating, bearing witness to, or failing to prevent acts that transgress deeply held moral beliefs and expectations."[36] As doctors, we know what our patients deserve but often cannot provide it because the business of medicine gets in the way. There in the garden, I asked myself: Could it be that doctors are also suffering from a kind of moral injury, caught in a conflict between the profit motive of our employers and our oaths to heal?

In his 1994 book *Achilles in Vietnam*, Dr. Jonathan Shay describes moral injury slightly differently, as "betrayal of what is right by someone who holds legitimate authority in a high stakes situation."[37] In healthcare, the stakes aren't always life and death, but for each patient, their health is always a high-stakes situation. In the first half of the twentieth century, most doctors worked in solo practices with minimal administrative support. Hospitals were locally owned and operated by the communities they served, guided by experts in healthcare — physicians. When doctors started banding together to form group practices, beginning in the 1970s, they hired administrators to keep operations running smoothly. But as healthcare systems corporatized and consolidated over the past forty years, most executives have come to see themselves as responsible not to physicians or to patients but rather to shareholders, who have one goal: maximizing profit.

Today, MBAs like Schoen control most of our healthcare systems. But there is one consistent face of medicine for patients: their physician. Bearing the weight of responsibility and liability for these profit-generating systems is breaking them.

For months after hearing about moral injury, I thought of little else. Giving up clinical medicine had been a personal loss, but now I understood the problem was not with me but with our healthcare system. I wanted other doctors in distress to know they were not alone, and for them to stop blaming themselves for their frustrations with clinical medicine.

In the fall of 2016, I shared my thoughts about this with my friend Dr. Simon Talbot, an academic plastic surgeon whom I'd gotten to know through his work in hand transplants and with whom I'd done other disruptive work. Over the next year and a half, we researched, revised, and refined the idea. Eventually we drafted an article about why moral injury, not burnout, was the source of widespread distress among physicians, which we submitted to journals like the *New England Journal of Medicine* and the *Journal of the American Medical Association*. For six months, we received only rejections, until finally Pat Skerrett, the editor at a new medical spinoff of the *Boston Globe, STAT News*, accepted the article. Since the day it was published, the response has been overwhelmingly positive. The article has been downloaded more than 300,000 times, and scores of clinicians — doctors, nurses, physical therapists, social workers — have reached out directly, telling us what a relief it was to have language to accurately characterize their experience, and telling their stories of peril. It became clear that patients and the public needed to hear those stories, and there was a growing appetite for change.

Before I started writing this book, I expected that physicians would be eager to share their experiences, but when I started doing interviews, it was surprisingly hard to find people willing to go on the record, even when I promised them anonymity. This is partly because physicians fear retaliation for speaking publicly about their distress but also because naming this problem would mean feeling obligated to confront it, something most doctors can't fathom doing when they are already working upward of eighty hours a week. I don't blame them for staying quiet; if I were still practicing in corporate healthcare, I probably would not have gone on the record, either.

It was, perhaps unsurprisingly, even harder to find administrators who wanted to talk to me. If they publicly admit that systems challenges are at the heart of distress in their workforce, they are assuming responsibility for issues they do not have the training, or the time, to address. Because identifying clinicians and administrators to feature in this book was so challenging, I am even more grateful for the people who did come forward, both those whose stories I tell in specific chapters and those who contributed background and perspective.

Even once people committed to participating, getting to know them well enough for them to tell their stories faithfully was a challenge. Most doctors have learned to hide their own pain; if they let themselves feel the extent of their distress, their patients might suffer. Usually, I'd talk to someone once, often for hours. Both of us would think I had the whole story. But it was only when I went back for clarification that I would get the real story — of anger, shame, disappointment, grief, fear, and the risk of being destroyed.

Some of the clinicians in this book are people I know from Carlisle; others I met through word of mouth, through friends of friends, or after reading news stories or journal articles that intrigued me. Medicine as a field, and particularly in leadership positions, is still dominated by white men, and although I talked to many doctors from underrepresented backgrounds, who confirmed their experiences of distress, most declined to be featured in the book; unless someone is in a position of power or has nothing to lose, speaking out is often too dangerous.[38] For the same reason, I agreed to anonymize three of the doctors in this book. And, of course, the names of all patients and family members, except my own, are anonymized to protect their privacy.

Every one of the generous physicians who told me the stories of distress and triumph that follow did it for only one reason: to make medicine better.

CHAPTER ONE

Timeless Principles, Changing Times

It can be tricky business when a doctor needs a doctor. Sometimes we know too much and want care from a peer with similarly high standards, or we want privacy where there is little. When I wrecked my shoulder working with a horse in 2007, six months after moving to Pennsylvania, I wanted both. After a couple of unsatisfying encounters close to home, where small-town medical and social circles overlap, I went to the University of Pennsylvania at the recommendation of a medical school mentor. Dr. Matt Ramsey had been at Penn for nearly a decade when he stepped in for his partner, for reasons I didn't fully understand at the time, to put my shoulder back together. At the first appointment, his waiting room was jammed, and he ran ninety minutes behind schedule. When I finally saw him, we discussed how to address an acute injury to one shoulder and long-standing issues from old injuries in the other. Unlike the previous surgeons I'd consulted and despite the backlog in the waiting room, he asked what my work, hobbies, and goals were. He welcomed tough questions, then explained my options in detail. But there wasn't a granule of sugarcoating in his assessment. He gave me the whole truth and trusted I could handle it. His recommendation was blunt: "Let's fix the acute injury, because at least that shoulder is salvageable, and we'll figure the rest out later." I left the appointment reeling, but relieved by his candor.

Since then, Matt and I have stayed in touch. We have talked often about the changes in medicine, how they are affecting the way physicians practice and our identity as a profession, and how to get out of the mess. I deeply respect his skills as a surgeon, but even more, I respect the way he approaches his work, and his uncompromising principles.

"Go to work, and work hard," Matt tells his three kids, an ethos he learned from his mom and his grandparents when he was growing up and which he models every day. As a clinician he is disarmingly direct. After spending years treating just two joints — shoulders and elbows — it usually takes him less than a minute to understand a new patient's problem and to plan a course of treatment. He spends the rest of the encounter getting to know the patient as a whole person. What motivates them? Where do they live? How do they work and play? What is their personality — hard-charger or bystander, rule-follower or rebel? He wants those answers in part because he can do a better job repairing a joint when he knows the stresses it will be subject to and also because he doesn't just care *for* his patients, he cares *about* them.

Matt has an easy confidence with a ready smile, and in casual conversation his banter is quick-witted and playful. But when he talks about his patients and his commitment to them, he straightens a bit, his jaw juts almost imperceptibly forward, and he's pensive, verging on reverent. He speaks of that promise as a reflection of his moral core.

In our conversations for this book, Matt often talked about the sacrifices he has made to keep that promise. For him, the hard parts of being a doctor are only partly about the work itself — the long hours, the physicality of operating, the difficult discussions with patients. He also grieves for the moments with family and friends that he gave up in the bargain. One day, he told me the story of yet another family gathering he'd been called away from and how wrenching it was to leave his daughter, still in pigtails, so he could care for a stranger. But to turn away from someone in need was unthinkable.

In 2002, Matt ducked out of the chaos of his youngest daughter's seventh birthday party to answer a call from the emergency room at Penn, where he had been an attending orthopedic surgeon for the past five years.

"Hi, this is Dr. Ramsey. Someone paged me?"

"Hi, Matt. This is Sarah Jackson. I'm sorry to interrupt your Saturday, but we've got a guy here who wrecked his motorcycle on the Schuylkill Expressway. Both his humerus and his scapula are a mess. I think he might need a little titanium and Vicryl."

"Thanks, Sarah. Give me a few minutes to make some apologies and I'll be in." Matt was the orthopedic surgeon on call for trauma cases that weekend, responsible for evaluating anyone who had dislocated, broken, or torn anything badly enough that they might need immediate surgery.

He found his wife in the kitchen refilling a fruit tray.

"Do you need to go in?" Nancy asked, her gaze searching for his. Even after being together for more than a decade, Matt was often surprised by how she picked up the subtlest cues in his body language. No wonder the kids thought she could read their minds.

"Motorcycle wreck. Sounds like it's bad."

"Go on then," Nancy said, laying her hand on his. "If you leave now, maybe you can get back by bedtime to tuck her in. She's so distracted by cake and presents, she'll be fine."

He knew his daughter would be fine; Nancy would make sure of that. But Matt was disappointed. He wanted to be there to help Nancy, to spend time with his kids, and to catch up with family visiting from out of town — his brothers and their families, his in-laws, and his mom. But not this year, and not the previous Thanksgiving or the Christmas before that, or innumerable other occasions. In every picture of his young family, he was either absent or asleep somewhere in the background. This was the life he signed up for, and that his family endured for his sake, but sometimes it was hard to bear that those he loved most couldn't be his priority.

Matt considered working in many fields other than medicine. But in the end what he couldn't resist was the unspoken covenant with patients. Every day, people submitted to his care, even if it meant enduring excruciating pain, based simply on their faith in his word that it would help. In return, he promised to live up to their trust with technical excellence, an unwavering moral compass, and deep compassion. He could not imagine a career that would ask him to be a better man.

Matt spent ten years training to become a surgeon: four years in medical school, five years in residency, and a yearlong subspecialty fellowship. The process transformed him from an enthusiastic, intelligent, but unfocused, young man into a principled, disciplined, and compassionate surgeon.

Though I didn't know it, Matt was at a crossroads when we first met. Over the twenty-five years since he decided to apply to medical school, the economic and cultural landscape of medicine had changed. Business interests — first health maintenance organizations, then large healthcare systems, and later private equity — were brokering the relationship between doctors and patients to maximize their profit from the transaction. Every year, he was asked to do more with less support — see more clinic patients and perform more surgeries with fewer clinical assistants and administrative staff — and his revenue targets rose. But there was a limit to how much more he could do without compromising the care he provided. And he hadn't sacrificed so much, for so long, to serve corporate interests instead of his patients' needs.

Matt was a curious kid and a hands-on learner. When he was five, his parents divorced and his mother moved the three boys from Texas to her hometown of Schenectady, New York, to be near family. His mother was a teacher, and although they didn't want for the basics, money was tight. If something broke around the house, she would tell the boys, "Have a go. If you can't fix it, I'll get someone in." She would often tinker alongside them to fix a leaky sink or a loose stair tread. Odds were, among the four of them, they would find a solution. With her encouragement, the boys developed resourcefulness, persistence, and a sense of agency in the world as they took calculated risks. When he later learned to diagnose and treat patients, the process reminded him of the problem solving they had done around the house.

When Matt's mother was growing up, Schenectady was known as the City That Lights the World. Thomas Edison moved his manufacturing plant from New York City to Schenectady in 1886; six years later, Edison Machine Works merged with the Thomson-Houston Electric Company, and General Electric (GE) was born. For ninety years, GE provided a sense of stability and security that is almost unimaginable in the community today; at its height, the GE campus employed thirty thousand people. High school and college students knew a well-paying, lifelong job with great benefits was waiting for them when they graduated, whether on the manufacturing floor, in a corporate office, or in the research labs in the suburbs. But in 1974, when Matt was ten years old, GE began moving manufacturing lines to southern states with weaker unions and cheaper labor. Every year the plant lost a thousand or so jobs, and those losses rippled across the community. Relationships frayed at the once tight-knit workplace as more senior union members bumped their juniors out of jobs. Pocketbooks tightened, so restaurants and retail shops struggled. People moved away, and real estate values plummeted amid falling demand. The community felt betrayed by a juggernaut looking out for its own bottom line.

Although his family was spared any direct impact, Matt spent his high school years watching job losses upend the lives of his friends. Even as a teenager, Matt was thinking about building a career that would allow him to provide stability and security for his family.

Science was easy for Matt, and he was fascinated by human behavior, interests that intersect in medicine. Growing up in the 1970s, television made medicine look like magic. Shows like *Marcus Welby, M.D.* and *Quincy, M.E.* portrayed physicians as brilliant diagnosticians and independent thinkers who thrived in challenging situations. The doctors he knew lived in nice houses, and, rare for Schenectady at the time, didn't seem worried about losing their jobs. But when

Matt reached out to them for advice, many discouraged him from pursuing medicine as a career. They told Matt that becoming a doctor had come at great personal cost to them, and they worried whether Matt's sacrifices would be worth it if someone else dictated how he cared for his patients. One friend's father finally told Matt his interest was noble, but that if medicine wasn't his personal mission, it would make his life hell.

Despite these warnings, he showed up for college orientation committed to a formal pre-med track, but the cutthroat behavior of others in the group during orientation soured him on the major. He knew if he took a long list of prerequisites — biology, chemistry, physics, calculus, English — he could pursue any course of study in college and still get into medical school, so he switched his major to political science, delving deep into what motivates governments and politicians.

When Matt returned to university after winter break his second year, he opened the door, not to the brash greeting he had expected, but to empty walls and a bare mattress. His roommate's partying had cost him his chance at a college degree. Matt was struck that a similar situation for him would mean returning to Schenectady, working low-wage jobs and facing an uncertain future. Previously laid-back about school, Matt vowed to buckle down, which was easier without the distractions of a roommate.

Shortly thereafter, one of his political science professors, noting his aptitude, encouraged him to pursue work with the CIA as a political analyst after he graduated. Matt was flattered but, in considering the idea, realized he wasn't ready to give up on medicine yet. Having paid more attention to political science than to hard science, he now needed to focus on both. Every year, there are at least two candidates for every medical school spot. To earn one of those coveted spots, Matt had to prove to the admissions committees that he was disciplined and mature enough to succeed, and grades were a proxy for those traits. A stellar science grade point average (GPA) was especially important, but every grade mattered. An application with a GPA that was merely "good" was likely to wash out in the first round of interviews. When Matt's friends went to parties, he hung back to study instead.

Why would a young person set themselves on such an exacting path? Even with the rise of health maintenance organizations in some regions, medicine still seemed like a good way to make a living. It was a career with tremendous responsibility and unforgiving standards, but great freedom and personal satisfaction as well. At that time, 70 percent of physicians in the United States ran their own practices, mostly small offices caring for patients they knew in some way — neighbor, business acquaintance, friend of a friend. Those doctors retained the autonomy to shape their practices to their needs and to those of their patients. Some physicians were banding together in physician-led groups of one or two dozen doctors; those groups hired administrators to facilitate their work, but not to direct it. Despite their protests of flagging independence and long hours, the doctors he knew lived comfortably and seemed satisfied with their work, which had meaning and served an important purpose in society. It seemed like a way to do well and do good.

In one of our first conversations for the book, Matt acknowledged that the stability of a job in medicine weighed heavily in his decision to become a doctor, but "it was never about getting rich — there are plenty of easier ways to do that." It is impossible, though, to disentangle money from medicine on a personal level for most medical school applicants. The debt burden of the education is enormous, averaging more than $250,000 in 2021, and if the career is a bad fit, translating medicine's skills to other fields is tough. If he was frugal and chose his work wisely, Matt might be financially stable in his forties. But debt would hang over almost every decision in the meantime — starting a family, which specialty to pursue, where to live, what type of practice to join.

He applied to twenty schools and traveled to ten interviews, all along the eastern seaboard. Medical schools use rolling admissions, so as applicants accept or decline, they send more offers to potential students. Months after his last interview, late in the spring, Matt was wait-listed at Georgetown University in Washington, DC. He was relieved that he might yet have a spot, though he worried how he would afford the tuition, equivalent to $46,500 in 2021 dollars. Then in July, the day before he was scheduled to join the military in exchange for a medical school scholarship, contingent on being admitted somewhere, he received an acceptance letter, from the State University of New York Downstate, in Brooklyn. Tuition at Downstate was one-tenth that of Georgetown, so even if he later was admitted to Georgetown, his decision was easy. The next day he paid his deposit to Downstate, declined to join the military, and took himself off the waiting list at Georgetown. At the end of August 1986, Matt moved into a run-down walkup in Canarsie, Brooklyn, across Jamaica Bay from JFK Airport.

His first day of class was memorable. After a morning of welcomes, at 1:00 P.M. exactly, a middle-aged physician with a bushy mustache and glasses, wearing a long white coat, a starched dress shirt with a neat bow tie, and polished Italian dress shoes, walked to the front of the two-hundred-seat auditorium. The chief of hematology launched straight into a patient's history and, using the Socratic method, chose students to suggest what other pieces of information they needed and what tests they would order to make a diagnosis. Finally, he rattled off the results of those tests and demanded to know what was wrong with the patient. Answers ranged from the mundane to the absurd.

Then he lambasted the class for ten minutes about the profligate, haphazard, ill-conceived workup they had designed, which ultimately came to the wrong conclusion. He emphasized how little they knew and humiliated some respondents, pointing out that some of the tests they requested might have killed the patient. In summation he noted that this was a cautionary exercise in recognizing ignorance, the danger it poses, and how humility, curiosity, stepwise investigation, and, most important, listening carefully to the patient, were essential to being an exceptional physician.

In less than ninety minutes that doctor demonstrated the wide chasm between how brand-new medical students and practicing physicians, with decades of discipline and training, approach a problem. The transition from college graduate to physician would entail meeting the exacting standards of experienced physicians, every hour of every day for years on end. Ingrained in every physician, relentlessly pushed to be better than they were the day before, is perfectionism in the service of the patient. Trainees' performance also reflects the quality of their preparation and mentorship — whether they fully integrated habits of excellence modeled by more senior doctors. Physicians are acculturated so that their conduct as a doctor is inextricable from their moral core.

For the first two years, Matt's full-time job was studying. As he recalled one of his professors saying, "The first year, you learn everything about how a normal human body develops, how it is put together, and what makes it work. The second year, you learn everything that can go wrong." The material was not conceptually difficult, but the volume was enormous, and it was presented at breakneck speed — just ten weeks to learn the gross and microscopic anatomy, physiology, biochemistry, genetics, clinical assessment, and imaging of the heart and blood vessels, lungs, and kidneys. Then straight on to the next block of six weeks to learn the entire musculoskeletal system, then nine weeks for digestive, endocrine, and reproductive systems, and so on. A comprehensive exam at the end of each block tested the minutiae of each system, because course leaders assumed students had fully integrated the basics, and the true test of their understanding was at the next level of detail. It never let up.

The most consistent bright spot during those two years was Nancy, who kept Matt grounded in the world outside of medicine. From the day he met her during his sophomore year in college, when she quarterbacked his flag football team, Matt knew she was the one if she would have him. He proposed at the end of his first year of medical school, and they wed and went on a brief honeymoon during the two-week break between his second and third years. Matt moved to Long Island, where Nancy taught at the public elementary school a few miles from her parents' home. She maintained her own circle of friends and shouldered most of the household responsibilities, a pattern that would persist for decades.

During the second half of medical school, Matt spent most of his time caring for real patients during rotating clerkships, with only a few hours in class for specialty-specific lectures. Illness and emergencies don't keep to regular business hours, and neither do clinicians. Teams of trainees — medical students and residents — staff teaching hospitals around the clock, every day of the year. As a trainee, "taking call" means staying in the hospital overnight, or on the weekend, to be available at a moment's notice when patients or other clinicians need help: Obstetricians deliver babies; neurosurgeons stop brain bleeds; orthopedic surgeons fix broken bones; internal medicine doctors take care of conditions like strokes, heart attacks, and diabetic crises.

On most rotations, Matt was in the hospital an average of ninety to a hundred hours each week, a typical schedule for medical students in that era. He left his apartment at five thirty in the morning and was lucky to get home before 7:00 P.M. Every third or fourth day, when he was on call with his team, he would work a regular day, then stay overnight on call, and come home at 7:00 P.M. the next day, thirty-seven and a half hours later. If he stayed awake through dinner, he was asleep not long after so he could be back out the door at five thirty the next morning. On the nights and weekends that he wasn't on call, he put in yet more hours studying for clerkship exams or reading cases to prepare for the next day. Once or twice each month he had a "weekend off" — from noon on Saturday, after being up all night on call, until Monday morning.

Those two years on the wards taught students like Matt about the incredible responsibility of being a physician. It was sobering to follow a first-year resident as they simultaneously fielded calls from a doctor at another hospital transferring a patient with a terrible infection; a nurse worried that a patient who had surgery earlier may be having a stroke; and an emergency room alert that a trauma patient was five minutes away and they needed everyone on the surgical team to help. Would he be ready to field those calls and manage those crises in less than two years?

Even low-stakes situations evoked a sense of awe. During a surgery rotation in his third year, an attending let him close the skin at the end of a case. As he held the needle driver to start the first suture, he realized the patient had never had surgery before. They would carry this scar with them forever. Even if the overall risk to the patient was low, the stakes still felt high, and the privilege of the patient's trust immense.

Matt started his third-year clinical rotations delivering babies at Kings County Hospital in the heart of Flatbush, an area that had seen dramatic swings in demographics in the 1970s, from the Italian and Jewish enclave of William Styron's *Sophie's Choice* to a majority Black and Hispanic population as the more affluent fled the hardships inflicted by NYC's bankruptcy. As a public hospital, Kings County was chronically underfunded and understaffed and relied on medical students to pick up the slack, from delivering laboratory or X-ray reports to transporting patients, assisting women in labor, and helping with trauma patients in the emergency room.

Always a visuospatial, hands-on learner, Matt thrived on the wards, where his skill acquisition was lightning-fast. He could see something done and duplicate it immediately with good fidelity, so he was given the responsibility and latitude he craved. During the six weeks of his obstetrics rotation, he delivered at least twenty babies under the supervision of a senior physician. Every single delivery, whether at 4:00 P.M. or 2:00 A.M., delighted him. He considered going into obstetrics until his next rotation, internal medicine, where he found the puzzles of complex, co-occurring illnesses equally fascinating. And it went on like that through his whole third year, with Matt easily imagining himself doing whatever specialty he was rotating through.

Finally, during his surgery rotation, Matt had an orthopedics elective. Right away, the specialty felt to him "like a pair of well-worn shoes." He made himself indispensable during those weeks, and in return, as the residents got a feel for his precocious skill set, they taught him the simpler cases they didn't need to practice anymore, and he took every case they offered. At the start of his fourth year, he did another month of orthopedics as an elective rotation at Thomas Jefferson University in Philadelphia. By the end of his second year at Kings County, Matt realized that as a medical student in an understaffed urban hospital, he had fixed more broken femurs than the senior residents at other programs, including Jefferson, had done in their entire training. He was building his competence, his reputation, and his résumé, all at the same time.

But just because he had decided orthopedics was right for him did not mean he was guaranteed to become an orthopedic surgeon. Orthopedic residency spots were competitive. He'd gotten the grades and national boards scores he needed to make the first cut. Now, with his application and interviews, he needed to convince a program, ideally not too far from home, that he would do well there. Another expensive, disruptive, stressful round of interviews later, he matched at Jefferson.

In March of Matt's fourth year, right around the same time he found out where he matched for residency, the Ramseys welcomed a baby girl. Matt was there for her birth and her first day at home, then Nancy's mother stepped in to help while Matt finished up his last two rotations in medical school. Nancy's return to teaching for the end of the school year coincided, out of pure luck, with the end of Matt's last rotation, so he was his daughter's primary caretaker for two months.

Exhausting as it was, he relished the opportunity to spend so much time with her, something he probably would never get to do again.

The acculturation of physicians that their work is inextricable from their moral core, which happens through medical school and residency, is an arduous process that, for many, feels like yearslong hazing. Over the past century, attempts to change the process have made surprisingly little progress, in part because the current system is so effective at achieving its goals. Physicians leave residency as highly trained professionals who function well under extreme duress — calm in the direst emergencies, walking repositories of reams of medical information, summoning good judgment no matter how many hours they've been awake — and who reflexively put the needs of their patients before their own. But that induction comes at a cost to the individual.

The model for surgical training was created in 1890 at Johns Hopkins Hospital in Baltimore by its recently appointed chair of surgery, William Stewart Halsted. Until then, medical school graduates, almost exclusively men, entered informal apprenticeships if they wanted more training in certain aspects of medicine, but there were no rules, requirements, or legislation to standardize the process. Halsted designed a training program of graduated responsibility and technical difficulty, according to a trainee's abilities, and he demanded they be available at a moment's notice, day or night. They lived at the hospital (hence the name *resident*) and could not be married. Dr. Halsted was an intellectual powerhouse whose contributions to surgery are evident everywhere today — gloves, gowns, and disinfectants to reduce infections; local anesthetic; and anatomical discoveries and surgical techniques that changed the course of the field. But his standards were punishing and his criticism harsh and relentless. From what we know about substance use now, much of his mercurial behavior and his prolific contributions to the field were at least partly fueled by his well-known addiction to cocaine, and later to opiates.[1] While the structure has been modified somewhat, the pace and culture of residency when Matt went through it would have felt familiar to Halsted's own trainees.

Because Matt was going into a surgical subspecialty, he could do his first year of residency, also known as his internship, at any surgery program, then join his cohort at Thomas Jefferson in his second year. He stayed put for his internship, at Long Island Jewish Hospital, to minimize disruptions to his family for as long as possible.

During training, workdays began before dawn with morning rounds, when the entire group of residents on a surgical team visited each of the ten to fifteen patients in their care, though on busy services, they might see as many as forty. The intern led the way, presenting a succinct summary of the patient's condition, any events that happened overnight, the results of every X-ray and blood test, the opinions of any other doctors consulted about the patient's condition, and a plan for the day. The team would talk to and examine the patient briefly, then fire questions and recommendations at the intern for more in-depth examination, testing, or treatment. The team typically spent less than five minutes with each patient, but the updates were comprehensive. Rounds finished by 7:00 A.M., so the team could get to the operating room on time for the first surgery of the day. The intern visited patients throughout the day, checking their status, conducting tests, and revising treatment plans. Later, the team reconvened for sign-out rounds after finishing the day's surgeries. The seniors filled in the interns about any tricky parts of the operations that could put patients at higher risk for complications, and interns updated the team about patients' progress since the morning. It was not uncommon for sign-out to happen late in the evening, and no one went home until it was over.

After a monthslong string of punishing days and brutal nights on call, Matt phoned his older brother. He was railing about how hard the work was and his frustration with being constantly criticized by his attending physicians. True to the Ramsey ethos, his brother interrupted him mid-rant. "Hey, listen . . . do you want to be successful?" When Matt replied that of course he did, his brother shot back: "Then shut up and go to work. The only way you're going to make it in the world is to buckle down and get back at it. Nobody wants to hear you moaning." Chastened, Matt tried to retort, but he realized his brother was right. It was also a reminder that suffering in a difficult job wasn't unique to him, or to a career in medicine, and this was a temporary situation. When he finished training, he would be able to create a practice that suited his needs and those of his patients, drawing pieces from all the models he'd seen in the attendings who oversaw him. His perspective reframed, he returned to the hospital the next day ready to dig in again and finished his internship strong.

The weekend after Matt finished his internship, the Ramseys moved to Philadelphia, and he started his second year of surgery residency, now focused on orthopedics, at Thomas Jefferson on Monday morning. Orthopedics was work he looked forward to doing every day, which made second year seem easier, though the hours were still punishing, and the criticism frequent and blunt. While residents today are limited to eighty-hour work weeks for safety reasons, during Matt's residency he was on duty more than a hundred hours each week; at least twice a week, he worked thirty-six or more hours straight. There was even a joke among surgeons that being on call every other night was only a hardship because it meant you missed out on half of the good emergency cases. Attendings believed that residency had taught them to function well under extreme duress, pushing aside pain, hunger, fatigue, and chaos when the stakes of life or death depended on split-second decisions, and it would do the same for their trainees.

Spending all those hours in the hospital, responsible for every aspect of patients' care, was physically, mentally, and emotionally taxing, but it also instilled a deep sense of ownership in their outcomes, as did the review process for any cases that didn't go well, known as morbidity and mortality conferences.

Every month, each department held its own version of these conferences. It was a way to learn lessons from poor outcomes and to reduce future errors of judgment or knowledge. The resident who cared for a patient with a difficult course would present the case in excruciating detail to a roomful of physicians at every level of seniority, then field questions and critiques. Attendings were protective of patients, whether their own or someone else's. If a resident erred because they lacked knowledge, they were admonished to study more and get better supervision. But if they erred out of "laziness," like failing to promptly evaluate a patient, the attendings took it as a personal affront. One such incident and the senior doctors would lose respect for the resident; a second incident might cause the attendings to question whether the resident should continue in training.

At no point in physicians' careers were they safe from this scrutiny. As a fourth-year medical student, Matt watched an attending tell a visiting medical student to pack their bags and go home because they didn't know the results of a patient's morning lab tests. During his intern year, he watched the chief of surgery ask a second-year resident to present the details of a recent procedure in which the patient had suffered minor complications — though the patient suffered no lasting harm, every complication was an opportunity to learn. By the second year of residency, trainees have learned that memorizing laboratory values and trends is a critical part of tracking a patient's course, so the chief asked the resident to review the results of the patient's laboratory studies. The resident recited the values incorrectly, then repeated his response at the surgeon's request, rather than admitting he wasn't sure. The surgeon, red-faced and seething, rattled off the correct figures and said, "Dr. Sanders, there is nothing more dangerous to patients than dissembling. You're done." Just like that, he fired the resident. As Matt put it: "It only takes seeing that once to drive home how central integrity is to being a good physician."

Not every attending was so damning with feedback. Some of Matt's attendings, like Dr. Richard Rothman, had standards that were intimidating, but they also took the time to coach as much as they scolded. Dr. Rothman told Matt that the best way to become an expert at whatever he did was to take a few minutes, after every single case, to think through what had gone really well, what had been sticky or awkward, and what he would do differently next time.

The intensity and duration of medical training was hard on Matt and his family. During the years he was in medical school and residency, his college friends got married and he missed most of the weddings. They had babies whom he didn't meet until they were walking and talking. Friends' parents died and he missed the funerals. For a decade, he was always in the hospital or recovering from being there. After weeks, often months, of being too tired to even talk on the phone, friends drifted away. It is hard to maintain close relationships without shared experiences, and there were only so many invitations he could decline before they were no longer extended. Maintaining some of those connections, and a life and perspective outside of medicine, was another crucial contribution Nancy made to their life together.

Matt and Nancy had two more children during his five years of residency. When we talked, Matt frequently marveled at his wife's strength, independence, loyalty, affection, and commitment despite the challenges of his years in training. He talked about how his early absence from his young family troubled him and how her warm, steady presence anchored the whole family. His life had been hard, but hers had been, too. It was important to him to acknowledge their shared sacrifice.

When Matt decided to subspecialize in shoulder and elbow surgery, it meant subjecting his wife and family to another year of hardship — miserly pay, no control of his schedule, no more available than he had been during the past five years of residency — so he could complete a fellowship, rounding out a full decade of education and training since college. There were only a handful of programs in the subspecialty at the time, but Matt felt if he was going to ask his wife to keep making sacrifices for another year, she should at least get to choose where they lived. It was a mutual decision that he would apply only to the programs in New York, near family, and in Pennsylvania. When he got into Penn, it was an easy decision to stay in Philadelphia.

Matt was only the second fellow through the Penn program, so he wasn't sure what to expect. Programs generally develop a reputation for the kinds of doctors they turn out — deft surgeons, strong scientists, and sometimes swaggering braggarts — but this one hadn't even graduated its first fellow yet. The head of the division, Dr. Joseph Iannotti, was widely regarded as one of the best shoulder surgeons in the country. His partner and fellowship director, Dr. Gerald Williams, had an impressive academic pedigree — he was trained by Charles Rockwood, a legend in shoulder surgery — so Matt was confident he would come out of the fellowship as a skillful surgeon. But he did not realize what a pivotal mentor and powerful sponsor Dr. Williams would prove to be.

Dr. Williams modeled and expected the highest standards of professional conduct. Off-color jokes, inebriation at conferences, or harsh words with nursing staff, though quite common in many fields of medicine at the time, were forbidden. He told his residents and fellows that they represented him and the University of Pennsylvania when they went out into the world, and he expected them to set an excellent example. In return, he was a powerful champion of his trainees, recommending them for jobs at prestigious institutions and suggesting their names for committees and leadership opportunities. In Matt's case, Dr. Williams offered him a job at Penn at the conclusion of his training in 1996.

Even with an ideal mentor like Dr. Williams, the transition from resident to attending was surprisingly hard. Matt felt like he had been making critical decisions about surgeries and had been responsible for patients as a fellow, but there had always been another surgeon who was watching over him to make sure nothing went wrong. He didn't realize how much reassurance that backstop provided until he no longer had it.

Instead of feeling liberated, Matt was tense all the time. He followed Dr. Rothman's advice to spend a few minutes reflecting after each surgery and planning how he might improve next time, but those increments were small, and accumulated slowly. He started clenching his jaw. Though exhausted, he slept fitfully, and lost fifteen pounds without trying. It took several years for him to stop second-guessing every decision he made and to trust that Jerry Williams didn't hire him because he was a convenient choice but because he was exactly the surgeon Jerry wanted as his partner.

Matt assumed he would spend his career at Penn, but just as he found his footing as an attending, the culture at the hospital began to change. Productivity targets increased, so his already packed clinic schedule was even more crowded, leading to long waits for his patients. Matt viewed running late as deeply disrespectful. He would have preferred to book appointments into the evening rather than keep patients waiting, but the scheduling system didn't allow that. And there were other problems interfering with patient care, from understaffing, which delayed his surgeries, to misaligned performance incentives, which led to infighting between team members rather than cooperation, to waiting weeks for insurance approvals for surgery or imaging. He felt stymied at every turn.

When Matt took the job at Penn, he was awed to be part of a vaunted institution, home to some of the best doctors in the world, and he assumed the institution would trust those doctors to treat patients as they saw fit. But ten years later, his mounting frustration made him think he'd been overly optimistic. Every day, the institution made it harder to deliver basic care with the dignity, respect, and compassion his patients deserved.

Talking with physicians across the country, whether or not they're surgeons, I've heard the same lament: They are working harder and harder to meet ever-increasing, always changing performance targets.

They're worried about what it's doing to patient care and to the close-knit community of clinicians. The sheer volume of demand is wearing them down, but their bigger concern is that they are breaking a promise they made years ago, when they entered the profession of medicine — that they would do no harm and always put patients first.

Later in the book, we will return to Matt's story as he confronts the threat of moral injury.

CHAPTER TWO

Profits Before People

"Dr. Becker, I'm so glad you're here. Can you please see Mr. Smiley? He's coughing up blood and I'm worried," Janelle, Mr. Smiley's bedside nurse, said with an unusual edge to her voice.

Janelle had intercepted Dr. Hannah Becker as she arrived for her twelve-hour shift at Fulton County Medical Center, an hour's drive from her home, through state game lands and over Cove Gap in south-central Pennsylvania. It was January 2021, nearly a year into the COVID-19 pandemic, and Hannah was the only specialist in internal medicine still taking care of hospitalized patients in this rural part of the state (though Hannah is a pseudonym, other details are unchanged). Her partners, one of whom was Mike Hilden, had been let go six months earlier, and doctors from other departments were doing their best to cover the service, but they weren't experts in managing patients with multiple complex medical conditions.

Hannah said quick hellos to the other nurses on duty as she dumped her coat at the desk, hardly breaking stride, and followed Janelle down the hall, fishing her stethoscope out of her bag on the way. As they walked, Janelle told Hannah how Mr. Smiley had landed in the hospital. Two days earlier, he went to his family doctor to get checked out. He was usually excited for the first snow, but this year he was dreading it; he felt too worn out to shovel. His doctor noted a soft heart murmur and shortness of breath, then sent him to the hospital for more tests and treatment. At Fulton County, one technician drew some blood and another took him for a CT scan of his chest. Then the care team diagnosed heart failure and started intravenous medication to get rid of the excess fluid. He should have gotten relief within a few hours, but after two days of treatment, his breathing was still labored.

When Hannah walked into Mr. Smiley's room, he was sitting up in bed, reading glasses perched on his nose, flipping through the latest issue of *Lancaster Farming*. Her sense of urgency dropped a notch — he was pale and breathing more quickly than she'd like, but he could think about more than just getting his next breath, which was a good sign. Then she noticed the bloodstained tissues spilling out of his wastebasket and the rose-tinted fluid in the urine bottle on the side table. Patients sometimes cough up frothy pink fluid when their heart is failing, but these tissues were stained deep red. Nor did heart failure cause blood in the urine.

"Mr. Smiley, is coughing up blood something new for you?" Despite her sense of alarm at his condition, Hannah kept her tone steady.

"Not really. It happened one time, a few months ago. But when it started again, I had trouble breathing. It got hard to do anything."

"How long has it troubled you this time?"

"Oh, off and on for a few days, I'd say."

Hannah politely excused herself, promising to be right back, then found the nearest computer and began skimming his electronic health record. After scrolling through dozens of pages, Hannah found a note from his family doctor a year earlier that mentioned a history of a rare autoimmune disease called Goodpasture syndrome. The words jumped out at her like a neon sign but might not have been meaningful to someone less familiar with the minutiae of internal medicine. Now what she was seeing made sense: An acute flare of Goodpasture would behave exactly like this, and it would not respond to the prescribed treatment.

Even with an accurate diagnosis, Mr. Smiley wasn't out of the woods. Patients with Goodpasture develop antibodies that attack their own lungs and kidneys, which can cause permanent damage and even death if flares are not caught early. Hannah spent the next six hours coordinating his transfer to a teaching hospital ninety minutes away that had the equipment and expertise to filter those antibodies out of his blood with a specialized procedure called plasmapheresis.

Mr. Smiley wasn't the only near miss that day. Ms. Lynch, a young mother with cancer, had for two days been treated with the wrong antibiotic for her pneumonia. And Mr. Miller, who worked hard to keep his mental illness under control, had been admitted three days earlier, the day after Hannah's most recent shift, after mixing up his medications, and no one had alerted his psychiatrist. Dr. Webster was livid when Hannah finally called him.

Until a few months ago, Hannah had worked as part of a team, so there was always an internal medicine specialist on call at the medical center. Handoffs between shifts were seamless, and the differential diagnoses and plans were clear and logical, based on shared training and expertise. Then, in the spring of 2020, during the initial stay-at-home orders, the hospital laid off her partners, one after the other, and replaced them with nurse practitioners. Hannah and her partners had always seen nurse practitioners as valuable members of the care team. She worried, though, that for financial reasons administrators were putting nurse practitioners in a difficult position — holding them responsible for diagnosis and management of acutely ill medical patients, without the fifteen thousand hours of intensive residency training physicians undergo. Now every time she reported to work for another string of shifts, the nurses were waiting with a list of concerns.

For the next three days, Hannah would review diagnoses and revise treatment plans, call families and outpatient doctors to get a better history or to alert them to new avenues of testing and treatment and arrange transfers. But she couldn't work seven days a week. On her days off, she worried about what would happen to her patients; when she returned, the cycle started all over again. Over the previous six months she had sent detailed lists of her concerns about patient safety to hospital leadership, but never received a response.

Sometimes it felt hypocritical to stay in a system that allowed what she perceived to be substandard care, and most weeks, it took everything she had not to quit in a rage. But Hannah was torn — Who would protect her patients if she left? She often felt like the last line of defense between her patients and bad outcomes. The nurses would try their best, but as the past several months had shown her, they could only do so much. And what about her own family? She was the primary earner, with a few years of payments left on her medical school loans, and her son would be in college soon. Hannah had worked for every hospital system in her local community and left when she could not practice as she felt patients deserved. The Fulton County hospital was as far as she could safely commute, given the terrain and the intensity of the work. If she left this job, she would have to give up her beloved specialty for a job as an outpatient internist, or she would have to live away from her family during her workweek.

Hannah's boss resolved her dilemma the following week when she asked Hannah to drop by her office on the way in for her next shift. "I'm sorry," she began, "but the hospital has to let you go. It's a purely financial decision, nothing personal." The hospital had already hired a nurse practitioner to take her place, who would be supervised by a doctor in a different specialty. Fulton County would no longer employ specialists in internal medicine to care for acutely ill patients.

Fulton County was Hannah's fourth job in a decade. She had worked for various types of hospitals — small community nonprofit, large regional nonprofit, for-profit, rural critical access — with each move seeking an environment where she could practice medicine according to the practical and moral standards of her training. In every situation, no matter the facility's legal status, she encountered systems designed by non-clinicians that circumvented her expertise or sought to extract more revenue from vulnerable patients. To Hannah, it felt like the oaths she took, to do no harm and to always put her patients first, were not priorities for the hospitals where she worked.

Hannah walked to a quiet stairwell at the back of the building, called her husband, and sobbed.

A friend introduced me to Hannah after they met volunteering at a mass COVID-19 vaccination clinic in Carlisle. Ironically, Hannah, an expert in complex illness, was looking for purpose and employment during a global pandemic. We sat for hours on my porch one summer afternoon in 2021, comparing our experiences of training and practice and lamenting the current state of our profession. She was struggling to understand how, over her fifteen-year career, the values espoused by corporate medicine had become almost unrecognizable to her.

Hannah's parents are German and moved to the United States for her father's job as a Lufthansa executive before she was born. She grew up on Long Island and spent her childhood traveling the world, with yearly vacations to visit family in Germany and trips to Africa, Asia, and Europe. Almost painfully introverted, she wanted nothing so much as to be unremarkable. Observing her new surroundings and adapting her manner to the local environment became as automatic as changing her clothes for the weather. The more she mirrored those around her, the more similar she realized they were, except she had been born into a privileged family. From a young age, she felt the obligation of that privilege and vowed to give back where she could.

Hannah remembers wanting to be a doctor from the time she was in kindergarten. She was always the child who felt others' pain and tried to ease it — the one who befriended the new student or invited the lonely child on the playground to join her game — and wonders if she might have latched on to medicine as a proscribed path to relieving suffering.

At Thomas Jefferson Medical School, in Philadelphia, Hannah still did her best to fade into the background; in her own words, she "melted away behind the gunners who wanted to be surgeons and tried hard to get noticed." She was in her element not in the pressured frenzy of the trauma bay but in the quiet of the medical wards, where she was captivated by the challenge of caring for patients who were very sick in complicated ways and needed someone who would do the deep work of piecing together the puzzle of their illness and their treatment. She fell in love with internal medicine and never looked back.

Specialists in internal medicine, known as internists, make up 13 percent of all doctors and fill various roles in healthcare: outpatient primary care, urgent care, hospitalist, nursing home doctor, among others. When Hannah was training there was a surge in demand for hospitalists, internists who care for patients only when they are in the hospital. Before the advent of hospitalists, most doctors worked primarily in clinics or small offices, and they had hospital privileges, permission to use the communal workshop of the hospital to care for their acutely ill patients. Patients, or their insurance company, paid separate fees to the doctor and to the hospital facility. In an earlier era, for example, Mr. Smiley's family doctor would have sent him to the hospital with orders already written for his admission. He would have dropped in to see him that evening or the next day to determine a course of treatment, informed by his knowledge of the patient's history, including that he had a bleeding disorder. This continuity of care was ideal for patients.

Hospitals hired hospitalists in an effort to maximize the revenue they could generate from each inpatient bed by diagnosing, treating, and discharging patients more quickly than doctors based in clinics or offices. Between 1975 and 2015, two big shifts drove a 40 percent decline in the number of hospital beds in the US.[1] The rise of same-day surgery with minimally invasive techniques and advanced pain management in the 1980s and '90s was the first shift. The second was the relentless consolidation of hospitals into large healthcare systems. By purchasing smaller hospitals, large health systems created a ready referral network to funnel patients into larger, more technologically sophisticated hub hospitals. But transferring patients to the hub hospital, rather than keeping them at the local hospital, reduced demand for beds at the satellite sites. Empty beds meant lower revenue. And hospitals that lost money year after year faced closure, no matter how much business they sent to the larger site. One hundred twenty small rural hospitals were shuttered in the past decade, even those under the umbrella of the most respected names in healthcare.[2]

This meant that the remaining hospital beds were in higher demand. Managing bed occupancy in hospitals is very much like flipping tables in a busy restaurant. If the lobby is full of hungry diners, the last thing the maître d' wants is a table waiting half an hour for their check. If the emergency room is full, and patients in the intensive care unit are waiting to transfer out to the floor, hospital administrators don't want those beds held hostage for hours until a private practice physician finishes their office hours and has time to write discharge orders.

So why not just add more beds back into the system? Just like in a restaurant, where more tables mean more space, higher rent, and more waitstaff, every additional bed costs a hospital $1 million when the costs of space, staff, and technology are factored in.[3] Better to wring more efficiency out of the current number of beds than to add more beds that might not reach a return on investment.

Some hospitals hired hospitalists as direct employees and could therefore control how they worked — who they supervised, how long their shifts were, what performance measures they had to meet. Other hospitals hired independent hospitalist groups as subcontractors. These independent groups were still their own bosses. They decided the terms of the contract, controlling their schedules, who they hired, and exactly how they cared for patients, but they were constantly tracking the regulatory and reimbursement landscapes, and the whims of hospital leadership, to improve their chances of winning the next bid for services.

Hannah had moved to the Carlisle area in 1999, right after finishing her residency. After working for a year as an outpatient internist, she decided she preferred caring for more acutely ill hospitalized patients, so she joined an independent group of internal medicine specialists working as hospitalists, Hospitalists of Central Pennsylvania at the nonprofit Carlisle Hospital. Built in 1916, the Carlisle facility was an imposing Georgian-style limestone edifice on the edge of the Dickinson College campus. Nestled between the college and the hospital was a neighborhood of modest limestone, brick, and Tudor-style houses, under a canopy of old-growth shade trees. Doctors, professors, businesspeople, and tradespeople passed each other on their way to work or on evening walks. Their kids went to school together and played games in the streets. The adults went to one another's dinner parties, exchanged pleasantries across wide front porches, and brought casseroles to ill or grieving neighbors.

That sense of community from the neighborhood carried over into the corridors of the hospital. The doctors called one another with status updates on their patients and asked for advice and guidance with complex cases. They knew most of their patients outside of the hospital, either directly or by association, so the care always felt personal. And that personal connection reinforced an already powerful, inescapable obligation to do the right thing for the patient.

It was getting harder for small, independent hospitals to survive, though. They lacked the leverage to negotiate higher reimbursements from insurance companies and volume discounts on supplies. The hospital itself needed major upgrades to accommodate modern equipment, and the board was skeptical the community could self-fund the project, as it had before. If Carlisle was going to keep its hospital, the board needed to consider every option, including becoming part of a larger system.

In 2001, the year after Hannah started as a hospitalist, the board of Carlisle reluctantly announced its agreement to sell the hospital to William Schoen's Health Management Associates (HMA). They negotiated a purchase price of $41 million, at the low end of its market value, but the agreement included HMA's promise to build a new facility. HMA's practice of decentralized management had reassured the trustees that control of the hospital would remain in local hands.

Hannah didn't notice a change in operations in the first several years of HMA's ownership. But opening the new $68 million hospital in February 2006, four months before I moved to the area, coincided with a shift in the relationship between HMA and Carlisle Hospital.[4] The first change was as basic as the facility's new, more expansive name: Carlisle Regional Medical Center.

The new building was a statement about where decisional authority rested in the relationship between HMA's central office and its hospitals and what the priorities were for decision makers. As D. Kirk Hamilton, a hospital architect, wrote, "The environment is at once the context for behavior and an influence on behavior."[5] The original design, based on planning meetings involving stakeholders including clinicians and patients, was to have only private rooms — evidence shows patients in private rooms have fewer infections, lower stress levels, and shorter hospital stays and are happier with their care.[6] Though this design would be more expensive, HMA leadership initially agreed because industry forecasters had predicted the federal government would require private rooms in new construction as it phased in the privacy requirements of the Health Insurance Portability and Accountability Act of 1996.

Late in the planning stages for the project, it became clear that the private room stipulation would not go into effect until at least March 2006. HMA's new facility in Carlisle was slated to open the month before, in February 2006, meaning the hospital wouldn't be required to comply. Without consulting other stakeholders, HMA leadership changed the plan from all-private to all semi-private rooms, thereby capturing the same number of beds for a lower construction cost. The last-minute change felt like a bait and switch to Carlisle Regional's physicians. "HMA promised the community a state-of-the-art facility," said Dr. Philip Carey, a pulmonologist who worked at the medical center during the transition to the new facility. "Instead, what we're getting is a hospital that will be structurally obsolete the day it opens."[7]

HMA also changed their approach to staffing. Rather than directly employing local physicians to staff the emergency room and the hospital wards, as Carlisle Hospital had done, HMA contracted with a national for-profit staffing company, EmCare, to staff those departments. EmCare pitched that their model of integrated patient care — staffing both the ER and the inpatient units with EmCare physicians — would eliminate typical bottlenecks in patient flow, because physicians working under one staffing company would seamlessly coordinate admissions and discharges. In fact, Hospitalists of Central Pennsylvania had always practiced according to this model of frequent communication with both emergency room and outpatient doctors, combining the efficiency of a hospitalist with the continuity of being cared for in the hospital by one's own primary care physician, but no one at HMA had taken the time to figure this out. There also may have been other motivations afoot, like favorable contracting rates for multiple hospitals. EmCare would consider hiring the doctors currently working at Carlisle Regional, but those doctors would be subject to EmCare's constraints. At the time, Hannah couldn't imagine going to work for a company like EmCare. It wasn't until she lost the job at Fulton County Medical Center fifteen years later and found herself out of options for work where she lived that she understood why doctors would accept work with a staffing company.

A year later, in 2008, the partners at Hospitalists of Central Pennsylvania went to work at Pinnacle Health, a nonprofit hospital twenty minutes to the north, hoping that at another hospital in the region not yet acquired by a large corporation, they would find the same camaraderie and support for patient-centered care they had practiced at Carlisle Hospital. They were quickly disappointed. Even though the hospital's legal status was nonprofit, the management principles were very familiar from HMA. The organization was buying up physician practices in the region, then pushing hard on productivity targets. Management wanted physicians doing billable tasks for 95 percent of the hours specified in their contracts. In theory, it seems reasonable that someone hired to provide patient care forty hours per week will do that work for at least thirty-seven and a half hours (which would give them a daily thirty-minute lunch break in a five-day week). But that expectation belies a fundamental misunderstanding of how physicians work. Patient care requires communication, care coordination, records reviews, and troubleshooting, which for most physicians amounts to roughly two hours of additional work for every hour of billed clinic time.[8] Administrators knew doctors would find time for non-billable tasks — even if it meant working one hundred hours a week — because, as internal medicine specialist Danielle Ofri writes, "For most doctors and nurses, it is unthinkable to walk away without completing your work because dropping the ball could endanger your patients."[9]

Pinnacle outpatient doctors and specialists were so busy they didn't have time to take calls from the hospitalists. Instead, their office staff took messages and relayed their answers back to Hannah. She talked directly to the doctors less and less often, which made care coordination and management difficult. Even some of the same doctors she had worked closely with at Carlisle Hospital, who sold their practices to Pinnacle, no longer had time to speak with her. Every minute they were on the phone with her was another minute they weren't generating revenue. The courtesy and collegiality that once made high-quality patient care possible were eroding under the pressure of productivity expectations.

In the meantime, farther south, Carlisle's patient outcomes were slipping. Some of EmCare's staffers were temporary employees who didn't live locally. They would come to the area for their shifts, stay in a hotel, and leave as soon as they finished. Their engagement was detached and impersonal, and the community felt the difference. Friends told Hannah that specialists were complaining to HMA that inpatient wards were like a black hole — they had no idea how their patients were doing once they were admitted, and the hospitalists felt little obligation to change that. After just a year, the local administrators at Carlisle Regional were unhappy with EmCare staffing because of how they were alienating specialists. They made the case to HMA's central office that Hospitalists of Central Pennsylvania was cheaper and brought them back.

For a couple of years, Hannah went back to calling the outpatient doctors to update them about their patients every day. Hannah's group hired a few nurse practitioners to support their work — putting in orders, doing minor procedures, making sure treatment plans were progressing and checking patient status. The quality of patient care improved, and both the community and the other physicians were relieved. But, unbeknown to Hannah and her partners, all was not well elsewhere in the organization.

In early 2012, rumors began flying around the community that an investigation into HMA was under way, but Hannah never put much stock in such gossip, so she was shocked when FBI agents showed up at her door in August and questioned her for hours. A few weeks later, they talked to her partner, Mike Hilden, and by December, Carlisle Regional was plunged into the scandal described in the introduction to this book. *60 Minutes* aired a report detailing allegations of fraudulent billing practices — unnecessary hospital admissions, payments to physicians in return for referrals, and inflated emergency room charges — at hospitals owned by HMA. The company would later admit, in a guilty plea, that it set mandatory, aggressive, companywide admission targets for patients seen in HMA emergency rooms, and at Carlisle Regional specifically: 15 to 20 percent for all patients and up to 50 percent for patients sixty-five and older, who were covered by Medicare.

The benchmarks were expressly intended to maximize revenue for HMA.[10] "HMA pressured emergency room physicians, including through threats of termination, to increase the number of inpatient admissions from emergency departments — even when those admissions were medically unnecessary," Assistant Attorney General Brian Benczkowski said in a press release at the resolution of the investigation in 2018. In that same statement, Benczkowski berated hospital administrators for interfering with physician decision making in the pursuit of profit — in other words, for causing moral injury.[11]

In 2013, Community Health Systems bought HMA for $7.6 billion. CHS was a healthcare behemoth, ranked 184 on the Fortune 500 list, with 136 hospitals in twenty-nine states and twenty thousand beds.[12] In 2018, HMA, which remained a separate legal entity after the sale to CHS because of the outstanding litigation, paid $260 million to state and federal agencies: a $35 million penalty, $216 million to settle a civil suit for false claims, and $62.5 million to settle the suit for unnecessary admissions. According to the civil complaint, which resulted in the $216 million settlement, "EmCare, at HMA's direction, repeatedly terminated physicians and ER medical directors who insisted on basing admission decisions and diagnostic testing solely on the medical needs of their patients, and not the corporation's profits. EmCare also terminated its own corporate managers who refused to coerce physicians to raise admission rates."[13]

In July 2017, CHS sold Carlisle Regional to Hannah's previous employer, Pinnacle Health. Pinnacle had been on a buying spree, purchasing four other hospitals in the region that same year. Then, in September 2017, Pinnacle announced a merger with University of Pittsburgh Medical Center, UPMC, the largest hospital system in the state. For its first eighty-five years, Carlisle Hospital was owned by a hometown nonprofit organization and run by members of the local community. In the ensuing sixteen years, it changed hands four times, including twice in a single quarter, and eventually became a tiny speck in a $23 billion portfolio.

UPMC took a hands-on approach to the hospitals it acquired: centralizing management, imposing uniform practices to standardize operations across all facilities, and hiring physicians directly. Hospitalists of Central Pennsylvania had to decide whether to dissolve their group, become UPMC employees and practice as UPMC dictated, or find jobs elsewhere.

Hannah and her partners had seen how UPMC behaved in other

regional acquisitions, so they knew what they could expect if they stayed. Carlisle Regional would probably start replacing more expensive staff with people who lacked equivalent intensive training — licensed practical nurses and aides for nurses, and nurse practitioners and physician assistants for physicians. Hannah's group still believed that if patients were sick enough to be in the hospital, they deserved expert care, so they parted ways with UPMC Pinnacle Carlisle (the hospital's new name) rather than submit to providing care that didn't align with their values.

From Hannah's perspective, healthcare systems were growing unchecked, and the bigger they got, the less clinician perspectives mattered and the harder it was for her and her partners to practice as they were trained to do. How did this happen?

US Steel Corporation was born out of the merger of Carnegie Steel Corporation, Federal Steel Corporation, and ten other iron producers on March 2, 1901. Founded by Andrew Carnegie, Charles Schwab, and JP Morgan, the corporation, worth $1.4 billion in 1901 ($39 trillion today), defined the city of Pittsburgh for more than half a century, its estimated value one-quarter of US gross domestic product at the time.[14] By its very founding, US Steel consolidated the steel industry. The next step was vertical integration, which allowed the corporation to take direct control of different stages of the steel-making process rather than relying on external suppliers or customers.[15] US Steel bought ore mines, foundries, manufacturers, shippers, and others until it controlled steel manufacturing from start to finish. But even a juggernaut like US Steel was vulnerable to innovation. The company, and the city of Pittsburgh whose economy was so heavily dependent on one sector, was devastated by the collapse of heavy industry in the United States and by the development of more efficient steel-production methods in postwar Japan and Germany.[16] It took decades for the American steel industry to reshape its business model and reestablish is relevance in the world market. But US Steel never fully recovered.

UPMC filled the economic vacuum left in Pittsburgh by the contraction of US Steel, and its rise was nearly as meteoric as the early trajectory of the steel giant. UPMC started in 1986 with the affiliation of three institutions, Western Psychiatric Institute and Clinic, Presbyterian-University Hospital, and Eye & Ear Hospital of Pittsburgh. That group adopted the UPMC name in 1990 and started its aggressive acquisition of regional hospitals and healthcare centers to consolidate the market. With UPMC leading the way, healthcare emerged as the engine of Pittsburgh's economic recovery. Fittingly, UPMC even occupied the US Steel Tower in 2008, gradually taking over more floors in the sixty-four-story skyscraper as every part of the operation expanded.

Vertical integration began in 1997, when UPMC set up its Insurance Services Division, "recognizing the efficiencies possible by complementing its provider network with a health insurance product."[17] The extent of vertical integration in UPMC is hard to fathom. Its healthcare delivery system includes forty hospitals, eight hundred doctor's offices, forty-nine hundred physicians, and ninety-two thousand total employees across Pennsylvania, New York, and Maryland, and it is the largest health insurer in western Pennsylvania. UPMC is also a teaching organization, training nineteen hundred medical residents and fellows each year and seven hundred nurse trainees each semester. It developed its own electronic health record, operates a human resources software company, provides health, wellness, and workplace productivity programs, and runs rehabilitation facilities and long-term care and retirement homes. Finally, it is a health research institution with an innovation branch focused on drug, device, and biologic therapy development, which receives roughly $600 million of government-funded research awards every year. The organization captures revenue from every aspect of healthcare, from cradle to grave, and bench to bedside.

This process of aggressive consolidation and vertical integration has been playing out across the country, with regions like Boston, Chicago, St. Louis, Nashville, and Dallas producing giant nonprofit health systems such as Mass General Brigham, Common Spirit Health and Ascension Health, and for-profit systems like HCA Healthcare and Tenet Healthcare.[18] In 2020, the smallest of these systems had 14 hospitals, employed 6,500 physicians and 9,100 nurses, and had revenue of $14 billion;[19] the largest had 185 hospitals, employed 39,000 physicians and 94,000 nurses, and had more than $50 billion in revenue.[20] Finding a physician in a small practice, who has time to nurture long-term relationships with both their patients and their colleagues, is becoming almost impossible, even in small towns like those in rural Pennsylvania.

Fulton County is one of the least-populated counties in the state of Pennsylvania. It is streaked, north to south, with the ridges of the Appalachian range, hemmed in by Tuscarora Mountain and the Scrub Ridge to the east and north, Rays and Sideling Hills to the west, and the Maryland border to the south. Until Fulton County Medical Center opened in 1950, a medical emergency — appendicitis, for example, or a difficult labor — meant a white-knuckle, hourlong trip along the vertiginous switchbacks of the Tuscarora Summit, then straight across the dozen miles of Cumberland Valley to Chambersburg Hospital, or a similar trip west over Sideling Hill to the small hospitals in Bedford or Everett, Pennsylvania. Dr. Edgar MacKinlay had sent patients on those white-knuckle rides too often. A Columbia University–educated physician who settled in Fulton County, he appealed to the Green Hill Civic Club in 1946 for funds to establish a clinic or maternity home in the town. The community responded by donating land, money, and labor, and the fourteen-bed Fulton County Medical Center, with ten bassinets to accommodate a busy obstetrics practice, opened in September 1950.[21] For decades, the hospital remained independent, supporting building upgrades, new construction, and improved technology through community fundraising, but the budget was always tight.

    In late 2018, Fulton County hired Hannah and two of her long-time partners. They had a solid track record of providing high-quality care, which led to shorter hospital stays, fewer readmissions, and more satisfied patients and referring doctors. All of that would benefit the medical center as government payment models shifted from fee-for-service models, which paid institutions based on the amount of care they provided, to value-based care, which staked payment at least partially on how well patients did and how satisfied they were with their care. The shift was meant to encourage focused diagnostic testing and collaborative, thoughtful treatment plans. The group had carefully considered what practice would be like there before signing the contract and were hopeful the benefits of working in a small community where they could establish close ties with colleagues would outweigh the strain of a long commute.

Before hiring Hospitalists of Central Pennsylvania, the medical center had relied on a patchwork of outpatient doctors with hospital privileges covering their own patients on the inpatient wards. A nurse at Fulton County for seven years, whom I'll call Jenny Wise, reached out to me through Hannah and said, "When Dr. Becker's group came in, our eyes were opened to what could be happening. They followed evidence-based medicine. They were on the phone every day with doctors and patient families, asking about goals and coordinating treatment plans. They knew when to transfer patients and honestly saved lives." Doctors in private practice who sent their patients for admission appreciated the regular updates from Hannah and her partners. Physician specialists' schedules weren't upended for unnecessary consults; when Hannah or her partners called, they really needed help.

But the type of care her group provided, as necessary as it was for the community, did not generate substantial revenue. To survive, the medical center needed to attract patients for more lucrative types of care — joint replacements, robotic surgeries, cancer treatments — which other hospital systems were trying to lure away. If enough of them went elsewhere, Fulton County might have to close its doors to emergency care, too, and those white-knuckle rides of the 1950s would return.

Hospitals find it hard to compete using the intangible concept of a "high-quality physician." It is easier to show patients the MRI scanners, digital mammography, and surgical robots that are ready proxies for quality care. Starting in the 1990s, hospital advertising focused on the latest expensive machine the hospital acquired and Fulton County Medical Center joined in, trying to remain relevant. It convinced this community of farmers — who would never think that each farm needed its own $400,000 combine to harvest its soybeans, instead hiring one for two weeks each fall — that it was essential to have a $200,000 digital X-ray system (in 1989), $1 million MRI scanner (in 2014), and $2 million surgical robot of its own (in 2021). While patients did benefit from access to those technologies, such large capital investments absorbed finite resources, leading the hospital to cut back elsewhere.

In the summer of 2001, the Centers for Medicare and Medicaid Services included Fulton County Medical Center in its "Critical Access Hospital" program, because it had twenty-five or fewer beds, was thirty-five or more miles from the next facility, and provided 24/7 emergency services. The hospital celebrated its inclusion in the program, intended to shore up financially vulnerable rural hospitals with higher Medicare reimbursement rates as "a major step toward insuring Fulton County's financial future."[22] For the first few years, the program worked and the medical center's financial position stabilized. Unfortunately, federal legislation in ensuing years chipped away at the benefits, and by the mid-2010s, the hospital was struggling again.

As with most health systems, personnel costs were the biggest expense. Over the past twenty years, the hospital trimmed nursing staff until there was no slack left in the system for a crisis or for someone calling in sick. Duties were reassigned from more expensive registered nurses to licensed practical nurses or nurse's aides. Administrators tried to replace older, more experienced nurses — whose salaries had risen over the years, commensurate with their experience — with new graduates, but it was hard to entice many young people to relocate to such a remote area, so nurse staffing was always tight. Though short staffing made everyone's work harder, Hannah's group didn't complain; they were used to working in those conditions, because almost every hospital in the region employed these tactics to some extent.

Then COVID-19 hit in March 2020, and Governor Tom Wolf ordered hospitals to curtail elective care — which accounts for one-third, or more, of revenue in many US hospitals[23] — to conserve limited supplies of personal protective equipment and to ensure that hospitals had beds available for the anticipated surge of patients with COVID. In the initial panic, and ironically at a time when the number of hospitalized patients was forecasted to skyrocket, administrators slashed inpatient staff, including Hannah's two partners, to try to stanch the financial hemorrhage. Fulton County was following the increasingly common decision among hospitals to reduce the number of physicians it employed and rely more heavily on nurse practitioners. Hannah was the last specialist caring for patients who were hospitalized, and she spent nearly every shift addressing diagnoses and treatments that well-meaning non-specialists had missed. She couldn't imagine leadership would cut deeper, but less than a year later they came for her.

During training, one of Hannah's mentors had told her that a good doctor could always find a job, and a really good doctor would never lose one. After four job changes in the past decade, she rejected that adage. All Hannah had ever wanted to do was to provide very good care for very sick patients, and she had just been let go despite doing exactly that. She almost regretted going into medicine in the first place.

Today Hannah is the only one of her partners still practicing medicine. She no longer does what she is most passionate about — taking very good care of very sick patients. Instead, she is trying to take very good care of nursing home patients, to keep them out of the hospital as much as possible, so they don't face what she has seen other patients experience.

Everywhere Hannah has worked for the past decade has forsaken patients in the name of profit and betrayed physicians trying to practice according to their training. The organizations were riven by need, like Carlisle Hospital; by greed, like HMA, CHS, Pinnacle, and UPMC; or by fear of financial ruin, like Fulton County Medical Center. The legal structure of the organizations, whether for-profit or nonprofit, has made little difference in what she's experienced working for them. They are all using the same shareholder primacy playbook from business school and getting the same tragic results. As a result of this misplaced focus, medicine is rapidly losing clinicians, like Hannah and her partners, who refuse to practice first for profits and then for patients.

CHAPTER THREE

Losing Connection

On a sweltering day in June 2016, nurse practitioner Mary Franco walked into the office of Dr. Don Kovacs, her longtime boss and mentor at Yellow Breeches Family Practice in Boiling Springs, Pennsylvania, and handed him her resignation.

"I can't do this anymore. How can my patients trust me if my eyes are glued to the screen? This isn't the way I want to practice," she told Dr. Kovacs.

"Me either," he responded quietly, his gaze shifting to the hand-written letter Mary slid onto his desk. With his left hand, he kneaded the muscles at the back of his neck, as if to work out a stubborn knot.

In 2009, the federal government had announced that within six years doctors would be required to switch from paper to electronic records, but the expense verged on ruinous for a small practice like Yellow Breeches — Dr. Kovacs estimated his cost at $100,000. For five years, Don and his partner searched for a way out of their predicament, to no avail. In 2014, they made the difficult decision to sell the practice to Holy Spirit, just months before Holy Spirit was bought by Geisinger Health, a system based in northern Pennsylvania known for innovations in cost control and quality improvement with ambitious expansion plans.

During negotiations, the dealmakers promised Don that he would continue to run the practice; Holy Spirit would simply provide the tools, like the electronic medical records system, or EMR, and the resources, like financial and information technology support, that would make his job as a clinician easier. But he quickly found out that those in charge of daily operations for the health system felt no obligation to uphold the promises made by their deal makers. To meet performance targets, Don had to change how he practiced: shortened, inflexible appointment times, documenting during a visit, seeing patients according to whoever had the first appointment open, rather than keeping continuity with one clinician. He felt defeated and betrayed by what practicing medicine as an employee of a big medical corporation had become.

Fifteen years before, Dr. Kovacs had hired Mary to care for teens and young women who preferred to see a female clinician for their wellness exams, because the doctors at the time were all men. The role was a good fit for her training as a nurse practitioner, which focused on managing straightforward diseases and encouraging healthy behaviors, for both the well and the chronically ill.[1] She always consulted her supervising physicians right away if she encountered anything unusual or unfamiliar during these routine appointments, and rarely saw more complicated patients in crisis.

Mary took pride in providing compassionate care. She knew the value of being fully present, taking an extra minute to follow up on a gut instinct with a thoughtful question, or just sitting with patients when they were in pain. During appointments, she would jot down quick notes and key phrases, then spend half an hour at the end of the night completing her notes when the office was quiet.

But since the acquisition by the health system, Mary felt like she had to split her attention between the patient and the EMR. Even when she was looking at her patient while she typed, the clack of the keyboard was a constant distraction and a reminder of her divided focus. And appointments were limited to twenty minutes as the health system drove the practice to almost double their "productivity" — the term adopted from assembly lines for how many patients they could move through the office and therefore how much revenue they could generate each month. She had grown to despise that word. It never felt like she had enough time or attention for either her patient or the EMR.

"When I saw Esther on my schedule, it hit me like a ton of bricks. We aren't interchangeable. We all know that, but the administrators don't care. If I treat Esther, when she should really be seeing a doctor, I'm afraid I might miss something and that she will get hurt. Our patients deserve better."

Mary paused for a moment, took a breath, then relaxed her shoulders and continued. "But I deserve better, too. I shouldn't have to justify taking longer than twenty minutes with Mrs. Franklin, and Ms. Saylor, and Mr. Jones because they'd just been laid off, or lost a partner, or admitted they were drinking too much, or because they're medically more complicated than the scheduler realized. I wanted to hang in there until you retired, but I'm not going to make it." Mary's steely blue eyes locked on Don's as he looked up from her letter. She swept away a tear as she said, "I'm sorry. I know this will be hard for the practice."

Don nodded, then cleared his throat. "It will. And it will be hard for me, personally, too. I value what you've brought to this practice and how well we've taken care of our patients. But I understand."

Esther was a longtime patient of Dr. Kovacs. Only five years older than Mary, Esther's six decades of poor diet, physical labor, spotty healthcare, smoking, and drinking had left her with high blood pressure, inflamed lungs, and liver damage. Two months earlier, she was having trouble breathing and called for a same-day appointment. In previous years, Esther would have called Yellow Breeches directly, and the receptionist would have worked out with the clinicians how to fit her in with the appropriate person. But on that day, she had spoken to someone thirty miles away in the central scheduling office for the health system who told her Dr. Kovacs had no openings and gave her an appointment with Mary instead.

Mary was meticulous and conscientious, but she was not used to seeing patients who were this precarious. Though she was well trained in holistic care — how the psychosocial environment impacts health — her training in pathology, physiology, pharmacology, and disease progression was less comprehensive than that of her supervising physicians. To keep up with the fast pace and increasing scope of care they were expected to provide, the health system encouraged nurse practitioners to rely on algorithms to make diagnoses. Mary had recently heard about an experienced nurse practitioner working in a big health-care system out west who treated a woman who complained of short-ness of breath and dizziness two days after surgery. She almost died after being sent home with oxygen instead of to the emergency room for a CT scan; doctors later discovered she had a big blood clot in her lungs. Mary worried constantly about making a mistake like that.

By rushing through her first three appointments that evening, she managed to spare a few minutes to click through Esther's chart. On the forty-foot walk to the exam room, Esther had to stop for a minute to catch her breath. Mary began the appointment by taking her vital signs, using those two minutes to observe which muscles Esther used to breathe, how she sat in the chair, whether she wheezed, the color of her fingernails and lips, and whether her skin was dry or clammy to the touch. She had always imagined herself a little like Sherlock Holmes when she was in the exam room — looking for minor details that could help piece together the puzzle of what was happening for her patient. But when she'd finished taking Esther's temperature, blood pressure, heart and respiratory rates, Mary had to turn away from her patient to enter data into the EMR.

The rest of the appointment was a race against the clock: She had fifteen minutes left to gather a history, review the details of Esther's latest visits and lab tests, conduct a physical exam, formulate a list of possible causes, explain her reasoning to Esther and negotiate a plan with her, order tests, provide instructions, and document every-thing that happened. The EMR also required her to collect mountains of data, in Esther's case her immunization record, smoking history, a domestic abuse screening, and whether her home was safe for an elderly person. According to the health system guidelines, which followed requirements from the Centers for Medicare and Medicaid Services, Esther could not leave until Mary completed the chart and provided Esther with a printed summary. Just doing all those things in fifteen minutes would have been difficult; doing them while also documenting them was nearly impossible. Going back to thirty-minute visits would have helped tremendously, but the scheduling system was controlled by the central office, not Yellow Breeches, and it was impossible to override.

It would have been one thing if Mary felt pressed for time with a few of her fifteen or more patients during each shift. But the EMR never let up. While she was physically exhausted, it was the mental strain that got to her: managing conversations, keeping patients focused and on-topic, filtering out extraneous information, trying to contain their anxiety and avert tearful outbursts that would inevitably slow her down. And this was with her normal patient load. When she saw patients like Esther, she was acutely aware of how much she might miss by having to rush her patients through the appointment. It was so hard and, Mary thought, so wrong. Her job was to heal, and that meant bearing witness to whatever patients brought into the exam room with them. But she also constantly heard the administrator's voice in the back of her head when he reminded them that their patient volume was low. "You could bump up your numbers a little bit," he told them at every monthly meeting.

Don stood up from his chair and stepped out from behind his desk. He gave Mary a quick hug, then walked her down the hall.

"Mary, you know this isn't what I expected when we sold the practice. We were taking such good care of our patients and running things so efficiently that I thought they'd be delighted to let us carry on. The only difference I anticipated was that we'd be completing an electronic chart. That was naive, and I'm sorry. The EMR has changed how we practice, and not for the better." Don let out an audible sigh. "I don't expect I'll last much longer here myself."

Mary Franco and her husband, Ed, a psychologist in private practice, live just down the road from my family's farm in Carlisle. A few days after we moved in, they rode their bikes over to introduce themselves. They had heard about a new doctor in town who rode horses and were sure we would have a lot in common. We became friends, and when I opened my practice, I rented office space from Ed. Mary and Ed had been in Carlisle since the early 1980s, when they arrived fresh out of graduate school, steeped in 1960s countercultural idealism and eager to help their community. I knew Mary loved being a nurse practitioner, and it was painful to watch her leave Yellow Breeches years before she had hoped to retire.

Don Kovacs opened Yellow Breeches Family Practice in 1978, in Boiling Springs, Pennsylvania, a modest farming community of about three thousand people six miles south of Carlisle. The name Don chose for the practice honored a nearby tributary of the Susquehanna River, world renowned for trout fishing. He had grown up and gone to medical school in Ohio, then moved to Harrisburg, Pennsylvania, for his residency in internal medicine. When he finished his residency, a nearby hospital offered him a low-cost loan and a guaranteed salary for a year to get him started in practice. In return, the hospital could expect referrals for testing and treatment when Don's patients needed a higher level of care. He liked the area, which felt a lot like home and wasn't too far from his family, so he jumped at the opportunity.

When Yellow Breeches Family Practice hired Mary, she had been a nurse for many years but had just finished additional training as a nurse practitioner. She joined two doctors and a handful of support staff in a very collegial atmosphere. Receptionists welcomed patients with genuine warmth and concern. The clinicians supported one another in every way, covering emergencies, discussing difficult cases, and swapping stories about their children. They cared for multiple generations of some families and, consequently, knew the ties, fissures, and stressors in the community — who was dating whom, who was fighting with whom, or who had just lost a beloved parent or sibling. Dr. Kovacs, for example, had treated Esther, her daughter, her ex-husband, and her stepson. They knew patients' medical and social histories almost as well as the patients themselves, and occasionally — though they would never disclose them — the clinicians knew secrets that family members kept from each other. It was the kind of practice the clinicians would want for themselves or their families.

For thirty years of practice, the partners at Yellow Breeches had kept operations as simple as possible. They worked from paper charts and kept scrupulous records, were selective about the insurance plans they accepted so their billing paperwork was manageable, and provided options to patients with financial challenges, such as a sliding scale for payment, or waiving their fees. They limited the practice size to keep office hours and after-hours call responsibilities reasonable for the doctors. Because they owned the practice and made the business decisions, they could control each of those elements.

The practice was not intended to make anyone rich. Revenue covered the costs of the building and paid staff reasonable wages, but the doctors had chosen good patient care over profiteering early on. The partners could have extracted more from the business by shortening appointments to see more patients in a day, reducing staff, or turning away patients without insurance rather than allowing them to pay on a sliding scale. They could have sold supplements that were of questionable value or offered cash-pay cosmetic injections to pad their bank accounts and to diversify their revenue streams. But those things undermined patient trust and clinician integrity, the very foundations of the physician–patient relationship.

Most of the excess revenue the practice brought in was poured right back into the business, to upgrade equipment, maintain the office building, or better support staff. The partners had set aside some personal retirement savings, but their plan, as was common for most practices until the later 2000s, was to build a well-run practice in high demand and sell it to a younger physician. The proceeds from the sale would supplement their savings and allow them each a comfortable retirement.

Don and his partners never expected it would be so hard to recruit a young doctor to join them. When Don went to the University of Cincinnati for medical school, he qualified for in-city tuition because his wife was a teacher in the Cincinnati school district. He left medical school in 1976 with just $4,500 in education debt, the equivalent of $22,000 in 2021. In contrast, the newly graduated physicians he met were mostly deeply in debt. With reimbursement levels by government agencies and large commercial insurers in constant flux, making income for small primary care physicians increasingly unpredictable, it was no wonder that so many young doctors balked at the financial risks of private practice in family medicine.

In recent years, insurance plans had begun requiring more and more information to make payment decisions, so Yellow Breeches had to work harder to collect those same reimbursements. Insurers changed payment criteria without notification and frequently rejected their first submissions, requesting substantiating documentation, like clinician notes or other test results, before agreeing to pay for higher-level tests or treatments. Sending the information delayed payments and cut into practice reserves.

Medicare is the largest insurer in the United States. Though not a requirement, nearly every other insurer in the country ties its reimbursement to how Medicare structures its payments to physicians and hospitals. Medicare payment structures have increasingly favored "doing" specialties, like surgery or interventional cardiology, over "thinking" specialties, like family practice, internal medicine, or psychiatry. Practices like Yellow Breeches were increasingly squeezed between higher administrative costs and stagnant reimbursement as other insurers yoked their payments to the biases in Medicare's physician fee schedule.[2]

In the early 1980s, managed care introduced the concept of prior authorizations, permission from insurers authorizing payment for a particular treatment. While prior authorization was initially reserved for especially costly care like surgery, hospitalization, or highly specialized chemotherapy, by the time Mary Franco resigned it had become ubiquitous. To get permission for just about anything beyond a simple office visit — prescribing medications, imaging, or referrals to specialists, for instance — doctors had to complete a form or call an insurance gatekeeper. Sometimes it took several levels of review and appeal before the gatekeeper granted approval. The doctors at Yellow Breeches started to worry about patients slipping through the cracks these delays created between assessments, testing, and treatment. Hiring additional administrative staff would have helped, but a small practice like Yellow Breeches could not afford the expense.

When Don was an intern, part of his job was to locate and review patients' old records to understand how their condition had evolved. He sometimes spent hours calling other hospitals, poring over reams of faxed records in barely legible handwriting, running to the medical records department, hoping the chart he needed was filed and not sitting on the desk of the last physician who needed it. He therefore welcomed the Institute of Medicine's report in 1991 envisioning ubiquitous electronic medical records. Easy access to his patients' records from care they received elsewhere would be a boon to his practice. What he didn't anticipate was how the broad audience targeted by the report would shape the EMR to their needs.

> We see it as especially pertinent for physicians and other health care practitioners; health care managers; medical record professionals; health services researchers; medical informatics researchers; computer vendors; third-party payers; the legal community; federal, state, and local health care agencies; state legislators; members of the federal legislative and executive branches of government; and, finally, interested citizens. All these parties, we believe, have much to gain from the success of CPRs [computerized patient records] and CPR systems.[3]

Over the years since Don founded Yellow Breeches, new regulations and requirements made billing increasingly complex. Billing codes, divided into complexity levels, reflect how much time, knowledge, analysis, and judgment goes into a patient visit. EMR vendors promised healthcare administrators that their systems would automatically remind doctors to meet coding and documentation criteria, resulting in fewer claims rejections and more prompt, generally higher, reimbursement. That got large hospital systems, and their lobbyists, behind the legislation.

Moving data historically stored in paper files into easily shareable and searchable digital archives could deliver powerful benefits to individuals, ensuring that the clinicians caring for them all had the same data, at the same time, without undue burden or cost to the patient of obtaining and transferring those records. Tests and imaging results could also travel readily between clinicians, improving communication and eliminating the need for redundant testing, which would reduce costs. At the same time, a large-scale health information repository would be a boon to public health, offering better understanding of health trends and the effect of large-scale health initiatives. By the 2000s, many sectors were clamoring for an EMR.

In 2009, President Barack Obama announced that the Health Information Technology for Economic and Clinical Health Act, HITECH, part of the American Recovery and Reinvestment Act, the stimulus bill passed to address the mortgage crisis of 2008, would mandate the adoption of electronic medical records. He explained his vision during his weekly radio address: "We will make sure that every doctor's office and hospital in this country is using cutting edge technology and electronic medical records so that we can cut red tape, prevent medical mistakes, and help save billions of dollars each year."

Passed in February 2009, HITECH earmarked $27 billion in federal funds to train health information technology workers and to help hospitals and individual practices set up EMRs. The mantra of policymakers was "the right information to the right people at the right time." Those that didn't comply by January 1, 2015, would see a drop in Medicare reimbursement rates.[4]

The easy answer was to install an EMR, but the cost for a three-clinician, independent practice was staggering. Don estimated the cost at about $30,000 per clinician, or about $100,000 in total. But the hidden costs were almost as much: a year of planning, project management, database improvements, mapping workflows, building dictionaries of terms, customizing templates, staff training, and reduced patient volume for at least thirty days before and another thirty days after implementation to accommodate the adoption learning curve. There would also be expenses in perpetuity for maintenance, upgrades, and additional security. Large healthcare systems had the infrastructure and the experience to qualify for and comply with federal aid. They also had IT departments, staff to support implementation, and more leeway to absorb changes in volume. Yellow Breeches was just too small to manage such a massive undertaking on their own, both financially and logistically.

While the practice was contemplating the EMR, rumors were circulating about proposed legislation, which would eventually become the Medicare Access and CHIP Reauthorization Act, shifting Medicare physician payments to reward value, rather than volume. While the shift should have benefited a small, personal practice like Yellow Breeches that had been operating like this for years, projections from the Centers for Medicare and Medicaid Services itself, contained within a 425-page proposed rule, outlined in table 64, that 70 percent of practices the size of Yellow Breeches would paradoxically see a negative effect on their revenue.[5] The CMS projections anticipated that small practices would face significant challenges in meeting the act's voluminous reporting requirements as well as the requirements for multiple specialties to demonstrate care collaboration. If the practice couldn't meet those reporting and collaboration requirements, they would be penalized with 3 to 9 percent reductions in reimbursement over the ensuing five years.

It was hard for Don to imagine how a $100,000 investment in an EMR would ever pay for itself with reimbursements slated to drop further. They were already running the office as lean as they could, while still being able to meet patients' needs, and their cash reserves were uncomfortably low.

Beyond the cost and onerous transition, news started to surface about unethical billing practices by large health systems that had been early adopters of EMRs. Just three years into implementation, in 2012, Kathleen Sibelius and Eric Holder, US secretary for health and human services and US attorney general at the time, sent a sharply worded letter to the five largest US healthcare organizations — the American Hospital Association, the Association of Academic Health Centers, the National Association of Public Hospitals and Health Systems, the Federation of American Hospitals, and the Association of American Medical Colleges: "There are troubling indications that some providers [hospitals, in this case] are using this technology to game the system, possibly to obtain payments to which they are not entitled. . . . There are also reports that some hospitals may be using electronic health records to facilitate 'upcoding' of the intensity of care or severity of patients' condition as a means to profit with no commensurate improvement in the quality of care."[6] Automatic reminders to justify upcoding were built into EMRs, but the owner of an EMR system was responsible for the accuracy of the bills it sent out. For a practice like Yellow Breeches, defending a claim of false billing would be ruinous. How would Don ever keep up with the regulations, legislation, and technology upgrades to ensure the EMR wasn't leading them into trouble?

Don held out until the very last minute, hoping a new EMR vendor offering a straightforward, affordable solution for small prac- tices would emerge, but in the end, with the January 1, 2015, dead- line looming for implementation, he felt he had no choice but to sell his practice to Holy Spirit, so they would pay for the EMR. After thirty-five years of being his own boss and the sole arbiter of what he thought was right for his patients, Don Kovacs became an employee of a large corporation.

The EMR promised interconnected communication and data collection across healthcare entities that would drive better outcomes at both a personal and a population level. Such access would have been game changing a few years ago, on a business trip with one of my colleagues, Steve, who suddenly started speaking gibberish. He understood my questions but could not talk or write a response that made a wit of sense. At one of the best medical centers in the country, which used a state-of-the-art medical records system, I spent an unnerving hour tracking down Steve's boss, who finally connected me with Steve's spouse, who recounted his medical history to the treating doctors. Truly interconnected medical records would have enabled the doctors to pull up that information in a few seconds, including a complete list of his most recent test results and treatments, from the health system in his hometown a thousand miles away. Then all the findings from this frightening episode would have been entered into the same record, available instantly to his own doctor halfway across the country, for coordinated follow-up care.

When Steve goes to see his primary care doctor at the local medical center, the receptionist doesn't greet him with any familiarity, although he's been a patient there for more than twenty years. She asks for his name, address, insurance information, and photo identification, then directs him down the hall to the primary care office, which asks for the same information and identification he's just provided to the receptionist. The same thing happens again when he's sent to the lab for bloodwork. It's as if he's a stranger to this system every time he needs care. Rather than the EMR re-creating the sense of Don Kovacs's office, where everyone knows him and his history, no matter where Steve goes for care, it seems to have had the opposite effect.

When Steve is in the room with his doctor, he sometimes wonders whether she would recognize him on the street, because they spend so little time speaking face-to-face during appointments. Most of the time, her eyes are on her computer screen. She'll ask a question, glance at him briefly, then dive back to the screen and *click-click-click*. Occasionally, she tries to disguise her distraction by asking if he's been on vacation or about his weekend plans, but he knows she's not listening to his answer. She's furiously typing while making the affirmative noises and nods he gives his long-winded seven-year-old. He wishes she'd just stop pretending she cares.

Equally uncomfortable are the occasions when Steve has seen her partner, who uses a scribe instead of typing for himself. A scribe's job is to be as unobtrusive as possible, to eavesdrop on the conversation between a patient and a physician, and to enter information into the medical record. It is a desperate solution to the additive effects of two difficult challenges: EMRs designed with too little clinician input plus too much focus on billing and productivity metrics that don't take human factors into account. The doctor with a scribe can look Steve in the eye and is much more likely to finish notes before the end of his workday, but the awkwardness of a third person in the room keeps Steve from being entirely forthcoming. It changes the dynamic to something less personal, less intimate, even less trustworthy.

Former President Obama acknowledged his disappointment with electronic records in a January 2017 interview with Vox's Ezra Klein: "We put a big slug of money to encouraging everyone to digitalize. . . . And it's proven to be harder than we expected."[7] Some blame the unreasonably short time line of eighteen months for implementation. Rusty Frantz, a Stanford-trained engineer and CEO of a top-selling health records system, said, "The software got slammed in, and the software wasn't implemented in a way that supported care." According to critics, the country's seven hundred electronic health records vendors, a $2 billion industry at the time of the law's passage in 2009, would have agreed to almost anything to get a slice of the $36 billion of stimulus funds.

With so little time before implementation, companies were forced to adapt software they already had on hand rather than building new programs with the end user involved in the process. As Dr. Eric Elster put it at a conference in Columbus, Ohio, in 2018: "The EMR is a cash register with a clinical note bolted on, as an afterthought." Many leaders of federal agencies wanted to leverage the technology — the Food and Drug Administration wanted to use it to track medical devices; the Centers for Medicare and Medicaid Services wanted to attach outcomes and quality metrics; the Centers for Disease Control wanted to use it for disease surveillance. The result was a rushed, imperfect system trying to be all things to all government agencies, with a laundry list of unintended consequences that mostly fell to clinicians to manage.

The introduction of electronic medical records interrupted clinical workflow, making it harder to systematically elicit important details of an illness and increasing the risk that a clinician might miss a key diagnosis. Notes in US EMRs are twice as long as they were nine years ago, and almost four times longer than notes in other countries, with different reimbursement requirements.[8] The bloat is driven by two things: to justify the billing codes used, and as a hedge against litigation. But it takes time — and close attention — to sift through the useless material to find what's relevant. Clinicians see the frustration, disappointment, and disengagement of patients when they toggle their attention between the EMR and the person in front of them; the practice also goes against everything taught in medical school classes about physician communication and expressing empathy.

While it's tempting to just ignore the EMR and be fully present for the patient, EMR documentation is a time-intensive task that would devour evenings and weekends if not finished during the workday. There are other reasons to enter the data during the appointment; many insurers, including Medicare, require doctors to send patients — like Esther — home with a summary at the end of their visit, which requires a completed chart.

Perhaps the most paradoxical and troubling consequence of the EMR has been how effectively it has driven clinicians apart from one another. For decades Don Kovacs had close relationships with the cardiologists, pulmonologists, and surgeons who saw his patients for specialty care. He would run into Esther's pulmonologist at the hospital while they were both doing rounds and ask for a quick opinion about a lab result or a medication he wanted to change. These informal interactions were quicker, more convenient, and less costly for Esther, because she didn't have to schedule an appointment, wait for weeks, take time off work, and pay an expensive copay to see the specialist. It also didn't overburden the specialists with office visits for questions they could answer without seeing the patient. But to qualify for the funds available to implement an EMR, organizations must prove "meaningful use," and one of the criteria is care coordination. Physicians must communicate with each other through the EMR to prove to government funding sources that they are coordinating care using the EMR. The simultaneous pressures of formalized communication in the EMR and productivity metrics that left no time for clinicians to bump into each other has led to clinicians working in isolation. The easy camaraderie between various specialties, even across health systems, has contracted, and relationships have suffered.

Although it never happened to Yellow Breeches, other practices have had to cope with the decision by administrators to cut costs by changing EMR systems without considering the effect on clinicians. Each EMR — because they are proprietary — has its own set of shortcuts, templates, and workflows. As one obstetrician put it, "Learning a new EMR is like learning a new language. It takes at least six months to become fluent, and during that time, my patients suffer and so does my family. It takes more of my attention and more time to do everything. I run late in clinic, and I'm more distracted. Plus, I take even more work home every night to do when my kids go to bed." Most doctors are salaried, so administrators don't have to worry about paying for these extra hours.

While the HITECH Act was well intentioned, its authors failed to fully consider how the healthcare marketplace works. Victor Fuchs, Henry J. Kaiser, Jr., Professor of Economics and of Health Research and Policy at Stanford University, cautioned in 2012, "I believe a well-organized health care system can benefit substantially from EMRs, but the fragmented nonsystem of U.S. medical care is not likely to derive enough benefit to justify the cost."[9] Because the HITECH Act did not require information sharing, healthcare systems implemented proprietary EMRs that amassed terabytes of valuable data for their own use — to advocate for reimbursement rates, policies, or legislation to help their bottom line.[10] Rather than operationalizing the Institute of Medicine 1991 report's vision of a digital record facilitating effortless communication and care coordination, EMRs have driven clinicians apart from their patients during the day, and their families at night, without substantive improvements to the care they can deliver, or the ease with which they can do it.

Ultimately, the pressures on Yellow Breeches Family Practice led to its dissolution less than five years after it was purchased by Holy Spirit and taken over by Geisinger. One by one, the clinicians left: first Mary, then Don, then his partner, each of them retiring years earlier than they had planned. After the final resignation, Geisinger shuttered Yellow Breeches Family Practice.

As I talked to Mary and Don, a quote variously attributed to Benjamin Franklin and others ran through my head.

> For the want of a nail, the shoe was lost; for the want of a shoe the horse was lost; and for the want of a horse the rider was lost, being overtaken and slain by the enemy, all for the want of care about a horseshoe nail.

The ripple effects of inextricably yoking clinicians to a tool, while simultaneously ignoring its usability, have been enormous.

Across the country, not just in rural areas, practices like Yellow Breeches are closing. The trend started before the COVID-19 pandemic, as practices staggered under the burden of EMR purchases and falling revenue and accelerated during the pandemic because small practices couldn't absorb the financial hardships of care disruption.[11] Doctors like Don Kovacs and practices like Yellow Breeches used to be the majority — only 28 percent of physicians were employed by large organizations in 1988. By 2021, that number had reversed and 70 percent of US physicians were employed by hospitals or corporations.[12]

For patients, the loss of these small, personal practices, committed to long-term relationships with patients, built on mutual trust, is intangible. It is simpler, in a corporate setting, to view employed physicians as fungible. But patients know the difference between doctors and can feel the chemistry in a good fit, which leads to better adherence to recommendations, and therefore, better outcomes. That sort of connection can also be healing in and of itself, and there are no metrics to measure that kind of loss.

CHAPTER FOUR

Dr. Sisyphus

When Simon Talbot and I published our first article on moral injury in *STAT News*, the healthcare community erupted in discussions about this new way of understanding the distress they experienced. "I *finally* have language for what I've been experiencing for years" was the most common refrain. A few weeks after our piece came out, primary care physician Stuart Pollack and two of his colleagues published their own article on the topic, "Healing the 'Moral Injury' of Clinicians Will Take a Village," amplifying the conversation and adding their own perspectives. Simon was excited to see that he and Stuart were colleagues at Brigham and Women's Hospital, so he reached out and over coffee they discussed how moral injury manifests in their daily life. "Moral injury is a bait and switch," Stuart told him. "We're promised that, as doctors, we'll have meaningful relationships with patients, and then we do so much data entry for our organization to get paid that the relationship risks becoming an afterthought. I don't want to think of my patients as afterthoughts."

In their article, Stuart and his colleagues wrote, "The health care system that clinicians imagined they would be working in when they began their professional training is not only markedly different than what they had hoped for, it is at odds with their internal sense of morality."[1] Just a few years older than Matt Ramsey, Stuart also entered medicine at the end of its "golden age." He envisioned a practice with the resources to offer comprehensive care, and the time to build long-term, trusting relationships with his patients. For thirty years, he has been trying to realize that vision: first, at a small independent practice;

next, at a midsized health maintenance organization, or HMO; and finally, at one of the wealthiest nonprofit health systems in the United States. In each of his jobs, Stuart eventually found it impossible to reconcile the revenue-generating demands of his employer and the greed of insurers with his oath to put his patients' needs first.

Stuart grew up in East Hanover, New Jersey, a town that covered eight square miles sandwiched between the Passaic and Whippany Rivers, twenty-five miles west of New York City. His father was an intellectual property attorney, registered to argue before the US Patent Office, and his mother was a special education teacher who founded a private school for children with learning differences. As he put it, "My mother raised us to make the world a better place by her own example"; already in middle school, Stuart saw becoming a doctor as a way to combine his interest in science and his desire to help people.

After earning an undergraduate degree in biology from Johns Hopkins University, Stuart stayed in Baltimore for medical school at the venerable University of Maryland, the fifth-oldest medical school in the country. For his residency, Stuart chose internal medicine because he relished the intellectual challenge of caring for people with medically complex conditions. He also had his eye on a career as a primary care physician, and internal medicine — among other specialties like family medicine and pediatrics — is one path into that work.

Stuart took an unconventional approach to applying for residency. He and his wife of just a few months wanted to live somewhere they'd never been, as far from the East Coast as possible. They couldn't afford to fly, so Stuart planned the longest road trip they could take and still get back in time for his next rotation, scheduling interviews along the way. Their westernmost stop was St. Louis, Missouri, where he interviewed at Washington University. He felt at home in the program and was thrilled when he matched there the following spring.

Internal medicine residency is three years long. Afterward, internists can pursue specialty training such as cardiology, endocrinology, or pulmonology, or they can start work, in an inpatient setting as a hospitalist, or in an outpatient setting such as primary care. Beginning in the 1960s, more internal medicine physicians chose to specialize rather than to practice in primary care; with some exceptions, more training led to higher pay. Over the next twenty years, the number of generalists declined, and some communities faced shortages of primary care physicians. Often patients would present their symptoms to a series of specialists — heart, lung, kidney, orthopedics — without ever seeing a primary care physician. Such an approach was expensive, inefficient, and sometimes even dangerous.

In response to this trend, primary care physicians began advocating that they become the "quarterbacks" of care, and medical schools emphasized the importance of primary care and preventive medicine, sending students on rotations in those offices and devoting teaching modules to that type of practice. Some new medical schools, including the one I attended, were even founded, in part, to increase the number of primary care physicians in underserved areas.

By the time Stuart was applying for jobs in 1991, insurers and policy makers saw primary care physicians as the key to curbing healthcare spending, which had been rising steadily for two decades. If patients visit primary care physicians for regular checkups, doctors can catch diseases at earlier stages when treatment is easier and less expensive. Once a financial incentive was linked to the vision of primary care as the hub of practice, with primary care physicians as the gatekeepers to expensive specialists, tests, and treatments, large systems bought in. Stuart was anxious to be at the forefront of this shift or, better yet, leading it.

For his first job, Stuart thought he might get the best of both worlds by joining a small group of independent primary care physicians in suburbs north of Baltimore. Each physician ran their own practice, like the old-time private practitioners he knew growing up, but they joined forces as a group to negotiate purchasing agreements and insurance contracts. The structure seemed ideal, but within a few months

Stuart became wary of the group's fast-talking business manager and a few of the partners when their assertions didn't stand up to scrutiny. Years later his mistrust would be validated when he learned one of the physicians lost his license for inappropriate opioid prescriptions dating back to Stuart's tenure with the group. When after a year, the collaboration he'd hoped for had yet to materialize and their leverage with insurers or vendors still had not led to increased reimbursements or reduced overhead, Stuart decided to move on. He was stung but wiser as he started the search for his next job.

This time, Stuart wanted a practice that had stood the test of time and had a good reputation with both patients and colleagues. His recent experience with a non-clinician leader, more focused on making money than making patients well, steered him toward physician-led practices. In 1993, Stuart left to join the Auburn, Massachusetts, office of the Fallon Clinic, a physician practice founded in 1929 by John Fallon and his father, Michael. They modeled their organization on the Mayo Clinic, where John had done his surgical fellowship with founder William Mayo. The practice operated as an independent multispecialty physician group until 1977, when the physicians in the practice, who saw HMOs as the future of healthcare, launched Fallon Community Health Plan, a regional HMO. The group practice partnered with the nonprofit St. Vincent Hospital to become the provider network for the HMO, which was known in the region simply as Fallon.

Auburn is a suburban, blue-collar town, ten minutes south of Worcester, where I went to medical school. When Stuart arrived in the early 1990s, he met patients from a wide range of economic and cultural backgrounds. For more than a century, mills and heavy industry had attracted skilled mechanics to the area, first from Italy, Poland, and Ireland, and more recently from the Caribbean and East Asia. There was also a substantial population associated with local universities — Worcester Polytechnic Institute, Clark University, and UMass Medical School — and a growing biotech sector.

The area had a gritty quality to it, though, with a high crime rate and a bustling drug trade. Auburn's tangle of highways ran through the middle of "New England's high intensity drug trafficking area," a miniature rust belt of cities where manufacturing had contracted, from Bridgeport, Connecticut, to Providence, Rhode Island, and to Worcester, and Manchester, New Hampshire.[2] Opioids were easy to come by and rates of addiction were already rising when Stuart arrived. His patients also faced plenty of the usual obstacles to maintaining their health — diet, smoking, alcohol use, sedentary jobs for some, and dangerous ones for others — and Stuart hoped the resources an HMO like Fallon invested in holistic care would improve their odds of success.

HMOs originated in Depression-era infrastructure projects. In 1933, Kaiser Industries, the construction company building the Colorado River Aqueduct east of Los Angeles, needed a doctor to care for its workers, and Dr. Sidney Garfield, just out of medical school, needed a job. Kaiser agreed to pay Garfield a fixed rate per worker, known today as capitation, in exchange for care when workers needed it. When the aqueduct was finished, Kaiser made the same arrangement with Garfield for the five thousand workers building the Grand Coulee Dam on the upper Columbia River in eastern Washington, and later for the thirty thousand workers at Kaiser's World War II shipyards in California, Oregon, and Washington State. During the Grand Coulee project, workers had the option to add dependents to their plan, and the prototype of the Kaiser Permanente Health Plan was born.[3] The novelty in this type of plan, unlike other insurance products at the time, was that it incentivized doctors and hospitals to keep patients well. Because payments were made upfront, if patients used less care, the health plan kept more profit.

The financial viability of an HMO thus rested on the ability of primary care physicians to engage patients in doing the things that keep them well — eating a healthy diet, exercising, not smoking, limiting alcohol intake, and getting regular checkups. Because it might take twenty years of a healthy lifestyle to lower the risks of heart attacks and strokes, a large proportion of an HMO's subscribers would need to stay with them for years to realize any return on their preventive care investment.

Fortunately for Fallon, the population in central Massachusetts stayed put. After its founding, Fallon quickly captured much of the healthcare insurance market around Auburn, so people could stick with Fallon even if they changed jobs. The population was also aging rapidly, and when people retired, they became eligible for Fallon's Medicare program. Between 1980 and 1990, the population of people over sixty-five in central Massachusetts grew by nearly 13 percent. The "old old" (seventy-five through eighty-four years old) and the "oldest old" (eighty-five years and older), who are most likely to be poor, live alone, and require assistance, grew by 16 percent and 25 percent, respectively.[4] These seniors loved Fallon's Medicare programs, which had a disenrollment rate less than 3 percent, on average, compared to rates of 15 to 30 percent for most other insurers.[5]

Despite its popularity, by the early 1990s, the organization struggled to pay its bills. The Health Care Financing Administration calculated payments to Medicare HMOs based on the projected cost for the average beneficiary, adjusted to account for local variations in medical costs by region; central Massachusetts fell into a low-cost category, which meant lower reimbursements for Fallon than for organizations just thirty miles east, in Boston.[6] But Fallon's costs were similar to those in Boston, resulting in unanticipated shortfalls. Moreover, Fallon underestimated the administrative burden of government-imposed regulatory reviews.[7] Lower-than-expected reimbursement and higher costs meant uncomfortably tight margins.

HMOs operate on similar principles to socialized healthcare, but unlike government-funded models, such as those in Canada or the United Kingdom, they compete for contracts against other insurers in the free market. When negotiating contracts, Fallon proposed the lowest price per employee they thought they could offer while still covering expenses and providing good care. If they guessed too high, the employers might switch to a less-expensive insurance provider and Stuart's patients would need to find a new primary care physician.

Though the integrated system shared risk — if there was a bad influenza outbreak, or more patients needed expensive surgeries one year, the whole system would bear a portion of the cost — Fallon Clinic was still a separate entity, responsible for physician and support staff salaries. It rarely had months of surplus cash-on-hand to ride out rough years, and floating a loan to cover those temporary setbacks was expensive. Because personnel are always the biggest expense in healthcare, when Fallon needed to quickly cut costs, it turned to layoffs. Enough bad years in a row and there would be no redundancy left, let alone enough staff to respond in a crisis. As a primary care physician, Stuart was in a double bind — every test or consult he ordered nibbled away at the system's margins and increased the likelihood he would have to cut back on support staff, but if he cut corners, he couldn't take good care of his patients.

During his first several years at Fallon, Stuart watched staff stretch themselves thinner and thinner, knowing that eventually they would reach their limits and patient care would suffer. Most of the time, his office had just enough medical assistants to keep up with routine tasks; unexpected crises easily overwhelmed the team, and they would run behind. Stuart's colleague, whom I'll call Dr. Vic Salvino, spent his five years as department chairman imploring leadership to increase staffing in primary care, to no avail. Fallon was physician-led, and leadership was sympathetic to the needs of primary care, but they just did not have the resources.

Stuart remembers the moment that moral injury came for Vic. It was a chilly October morning in 2003, shortly after he replaced Vic as chair of internal medicine, and the primary care team was meeting with department administrators in a cluttered, windowless conference room. What stuck with Stuart, even years later, was the banality of the moment Vic broke.

The radiology department had good news. After months of work, everything was in place so that a woman with an abnormal finding on her routine mammogram could get a biopsy the same day, rather than waiting weeks to find out if she had cancer. They were meeting that day to discuss whether the radiologist or the patient's primary care physician would notify her about the results of the biopsy, in the event of bad news. The radiologists were under pressure to read as many studies as possible, and the consensus in the room was that the radiologists were less practiced at talking to patients, let alone communicating a life-changing diagnosis like cancer. But the primary care physicians already stayed late into the evening almost every day to finish their notes and to respond to patient concerns by phone or email. They couldn't imagine adding one more responsibility to their overbooked days.

James, one of the young clinic administrators, chimed in, trying to be helpful: "This is the last step we need to put in place to start this service. Does anyone have thoughts about how to manage the workflow for these notifications?"

"Look, I can't take on one more thing, and I don't think anyone else on my team can either," said Vic, straightening his coat and leaning back from the table. "I don't like what I'm about to say," he continued, "but I don't have any other solutions. A nurse navigator would still hit the budget, but not as hard. I think we should hire one to make the calls."

Vic rested his folded hands on the notebook open in front of him. He sat uncharacteristically still, staring down at the table, his head bowed. After an uncomfortable half minute, he took a deep breath and raised his head, meeting James's gaze.

"Can you make that happen?"

"I will do my best," James replied, wondering how the idea would go over with his boss. Adding a nurse would be a significant expense no one had considered when planning this initiative.

Vic pushed his chair back from the conference room table and sat for a moment, slumped in his seat.

"Stuart, you've heard my piece. I have patients to see," Vic said softly. Then he left the meeting early, before he could hear James explain how they would implement the new plan.

Stuart was stunned. This meeting was the culmination of six months of negotiations about improving care for patients. Hearing Vic relinquish what he had always told Stuart was the most important part of his job — the strong relationship with his patients that would see them through dark times — was devastating. Stuart didn't imagine he was a better physician, or a better man, than Vic. What would happen to him if he stayed in medicine but, like Vic, was perpetually frustrated by a system where the relationships central to good primary care were squeezed out of every interaction by the business imperatives of the organization?

Dr. Salvino's tenure had followed a familiar pattern, one Stuart and his colleagues had seen play out a few times. A physician would take on the role of department chair, acting as the liaison between the administrative leadership and clinicians. After five years of doing a thankless job, trying to negotiate additional resources for the department and failing, the exasperated, exhausted leader would give up, and a younger physician would step up to the position, still optimistic that administrators might listen to the primary care physicians who were supposed to be at the heart of the health system.

Not long before that meeting, Vic had stepped down, and he recommended that Stuart replace him as chair. Despite his ambivalence, having seen what Vic went through, Stuart took on the role. Someone had to stand up for their patients and the physicians taking care of them. But despite fighting as hard and as smart as he could, Stuart never got approval for his department to hire that nurse navigator. For the sake of their patients, the primary care physicians ended up extending their already long days and making the phone calls.

During his four and a half years as chair, Stuart left his house every weekday at six in the morning and almost never came home without several more hours of work to do that evening. He would grab a quick dinner with his family, then head to his computer and bury himself in unfinished notes until bedtime. At his wife's insistence, Stuart took Saturdays off, and four weeks each year, they took family vacations, but the remaining forty-eight weeks were marathons. Meeting his obligations to his patients, his colleagues, and his family took all his energy. He stopped exercising for lack of time and ate junk food when he was stressed, things he counseled his patients against with newfound empathy as his own waistline expanded. He wasn't sure how much longer he could keep up this pace.

In 2007, his son started applying to college, and Stuart, no longer worried about uprooting his son, started looking for a different job. Fallon served its community as well as it could, within the constraints of its funding, but Stuart had almost twenty years before he expected to retire, and he still hoped to find an environment that could support his vision for primary care. He was also troubled by the dwindling number of residents choosing to go into primary care, and he hoped to inspire more doctors to enter the field. Stuart focused his search on large, well-resourced systems associated with a medical school. His model practice would need subsidies to have a shot at success, since insurance reimbursements alone would never cover allocating so many resources for primary care.

Soon he was negotiating his dream job at Harvard's Brigham and Women's Hospital in Boston. Brigham hired Stuart to design and lead his ultimate primary care practice: a multidisciplinary team, co-located in one office, aligned with patients' identified goals and wishes, connected through the electronic medical record and the Brigham network of specialists. Brigham called this model of holistic care a "medical home." If Stuart succeeded, his clinic could serve as a model for medical homes nationwide.

In the summer of 2008, Stuart cleared out his office at Fallon and moved forty-five miles east to Boston to begin developing the medical home model for Brigham. Brigham is part of Mass General Brigham, a sprawling healthcare system centered on two flagship hospitals — Massachusetts General and Brigham and Women's — in downtown Boston. Twelve smaller hospitals across the state are part of the organization, which counts seven thousand physicians among its seventy-four thousand employees. Mass General Brigham has net assets of nearly $14 billion — making it one of the five wealthiest nonprofit health systems in the United States — and an annual research budget of nearly $2 billion.[8] Like the University of Pittsburgh Medical Center discussed in chapter 2, it is vertically and horizontally consolidated, with hospital and physician networks, community health centers, home health agencies, and an insurer.

Stuart spent thirty hours per week treating patients in an outpatient office thirty miles southwest of Boston in Foxborough, Massachusetts, best known as the home of the New England Patriots football team, and dedicated the rest of his time to developing a pilot program of total clinical care for South Huntington, a new site in Boston. He would have more than double the level of support he had at Fallon: physician assistants, nurses, social workers, a pharmacist, a nutritionist, a population manager, and a community resource manager. For the first time, Stuart could serve most of his patients' needs in one place, including challenges like behavioral health, medication access, transportation, housing, and food insecurity.

One of the reasons Brigham supported the project was to stay on the cutting edge, since medical homes were considered an innovative model for primary care. The other reason was financial. The group designing the medical home anticipated that within a few years, the majority of Medicare reimbursement would shift from fee-for-service to a value-based care model. Because most commercial insurers mirrored Medicare's payment structures, Brigham expected them to shift, too. Soon quality and outcomes of care would determine reimbursements, rather than the quantity of services rendered, and investing in comprehensive primary care would finally make financial sense.

After three years of planning, Stuart opened the South Huntington office in 2011. For the first few years of the new practice, panel sizes, or the number of patients served by each physician in the pilot program, were small, and resources matched patient needs. For the first time, Stuart practiced as he imagined he would when he went to medical school. He took time to ask patients about who they were, not just what was troubling them. When a patient disclosed their challenges — with mental health, medication access, or food insecurity — he guided them immediately to a team member who could help. He even managed to make house calls on occasion when his patients became homebound. The team talked about their patients more as the people they were rather than the diseases they suffered — Mr. Jones the gardener rather than Mr. Jones with emphysema and diabetes. It was intensely satisfying to see that his vision made a difference in how his patients experienced their care and how his colleagues felt about their work.

In one of our conversations, Stuart told me about a patient from his first year running the medical home who had a devastating form of dementia and was declining rapidly. The patient's wife was over-whelmed and demanding with the team, but instead of reducing their contact as many offices might have done, Stuart increased their visits to provide additional support. When it became too difficult for the couple to come into the office, he made house calls. And when his patient died at home at two o'clock in the morning, Stuart got up, dressed as if he were going into the office, and paid one last visit. "If she could care for him twenty-four hours a day for months, I could get up one time at two in the morning and not hand them over to strangers, like the police or the fire department," he reflected. "Surely I could do one hard thing when she'd done so many." At Fallon, Stuart would have struggled to fit this patient in more frequently, and he would not have been able to make house calls. His schedule was booked weeks out, and his colleagues and support staff were too busy to cover his practice during the hours he would be at a patient's home. It was a relief to finally care for patients in a more holistic way.

Brigham heavily subsidized Stuart's initiative with pooled resources from across the organization. Stuart knew that altruism was not behind those contributions. Other departments, especially the highly lucrative, procedure-based ones, were still operating in a fee-for-service payment system. They agreed to subsidize primary care because the downstream revenue — from imaging, laboratory studies, specialist referrals, and especially the emergency room and hospital admissions — would be two to three times the size of their subsidy, a phenomenon some primary care physicians refer to as "feeding the beast." But that led to something of a conundrum for Stuart, since the goal of his program was to develop a value-based model that kept patients healthier, and therefore in need of fewer tests and specialist appointments.[9]

Early results showed the practice performed in line with most early medical homes, decreasing emergency room visits and preventable hospitalizations by one-third. In an academic medical system, where available beds are always scarce, preventing low-margin admissions keeps beds open for high-profit, high-tech, procedural admissions. The volume of specialty referrals did not change, because while Stuart and his colleagues did identify diseases at earlier stages, when they could be treated by the primary care physician, they also caught many untreated conditions in their patients who had delayed care, or who hadn't ever had such close attention to their care.

In what seemed like serendipity to Stuart, three months after the practice opened, Brigham became one of the first Medicare Pioneer accountable care organizations. Accountable care organizations allow doctors and patients to decide on good care and reward organizations that deliver high-quality care with bonuses. Moreover, costs are shared among the contracted organizations — insurer and hospital or clinician — rather than each billing separately for their services. Stuart expected that these bonuses would increase funding for the medical home, so they could expand services, or add staff as the practice grew, without depending so heavily on other departments for subsidies.

As word spread, though, more patients joined the program, and within a few years, panel sizes had nearly doubled, with each physician responsible for about two thousand patients. The volume of calls and emails his team fielded every day was staggering. They were doing amazing work, and taking very good, comprehensive care of their patients, but it came at a cost to their well-being. His staff were constantly faced with deciding whose needs took priority — theirs, to catch their breath, refocus their attention, grab a quick bite to eat, or leave the office in time to pick up kids — or their patients', and because of how they were trained, it was always patient needs first.

Every year when Stuart's division submitted their budget to the department of medicine and the hospital, they requested more team members to meet the demands of growing panels, but they received only a small percentage of their request — say, three new staff across forty offices. The primary care staff were stretched too thin, and it was taking a toll. Though he sometimes had the funds to hire additional clinicians, as soon as Brigham brought in new people, others would leave or cut down to part-time. Support staff also started leaving, for less stressful jobs in other specialties or to walk away from healthcare altogether. And the residents who started training intent on practicing primary care watched what was happening and instead became hospitalists or specialists.

Six years into his time at Brigham, and three years after becoming an accountable care organization, Stuart was bitterly disappointed in his employer. The Advanced Primary Care team was delivering outstanding care, so Brigham always qualified for a bonus, but when the money arrived, it went straight to Mass General Brigham's central business office. As it trickled down through the layers of the organization on its way to Stuart's team — from the health system comptroller to the hospital, then to the department of medicine, then the division of primary care — each layer took a cut. By the time it got to Stuart and his team, it was a sliver of the millions his team had earned, and it wasn't enough to support more staff.

Stuart contemplated capping the number of patients in the practice, which at least would keep the workload from getting much worse. But access to primary care in Boston was already limited, and the group had promised to take care of as many patients from the community as possible.

After three decades as a primary care physician, Stuart felt betrayed — by society, which puts just 6 percent of total healthcare spending toward primary care but expects those clinicians to address not just medical issues, which are enough in themselves, but also food and housing insecurity, domestic violence, and the inequities of underserved populations; by the government and private employers, who pay for most healthcare but whose policies and practices erode the profession he loves; by insurers who expect him to care for patients every hour of every day but only pay for in-person visits done by him, not by other members of the care team, and not for phone calls or emails or texts, as if the latter don't take time or expertise; and by an organization that has the financial resources, but not the will, to push back against the payers and insurers to build a healthcare system that supports the relationships that he, his team, and his patients value so much. Would it ever be possible to provide high-quality care in a way that was sustainable for his team?

When I met Stuart in 2021, he had been at Brigham for twelve years. The medical home program was meeting its targets for growth and patient satisfaction, and Brigham supported expanding it. But Stuart despaired at the toll the workload was taking on the clinicians who worked there and how powerless he was to do anything about it. Even his most committed support staff were losing hope that the work might relent, and each resignation was a punch to the gut for Stuart. Though he was nearing the end of his career, he wasn't ready to retire, and building a practice elsewhere didn't make sense. But to stay in medicine, something had to give. Talking with Stuart in the spring of 2022, he planned to step down from his leadership positions within six months. He was looking forward to going back to his professional roots and working half-time in the clinic without administrative responsibilities and a panel capped at nine hundred patients. "I'm not giving up on my patients," he reflected. "I'm giving up on fixing things."

During one of our conversations, Stuart confessed feeling guilty that primary care as a field is in worse shape today than it was when he became chair of medicine at Fallon eighteen years ago. "Sometimes I wonder if I've really succeeded at anything," he told me. "We take great care of our patients, but I haven't been able to take equally good care of my staff, no matter how many ways I've tried. Being a primary care physician is the best job in the world, but only when you have the resources you need to get it done. That leaves two choices. You can take care of fewer patients, meaning that primary care becomes a luxury for those who can afford it, instead of a right for everyone. Or you can double the size of the primary care teams, which has always been my answer, but never seemed to happen." Listening to him, I thought of the myth of Sisyphus, forever pushing a rock up a hill only for it to roll back down.

Stuart's dilemma is familiar to many doctors. They feel complicit in some form of moral injury, but they can't see any way around it if they plan to keep practicing. Staying in medicine, fully aware of this conflict, can be unbearably painful. Jennifer Freyd is a psychologist at the University of Oregon who writes about a phenomenon she calls "betrayal blindness," in which people remain unconscious of certain interpersonal or organizational dynamics to avoid recognizing treachery or injustice.[10] In the context of medicine, betrayal blindness allows doctors to protect their view of themselves as good people doing good work, rather than participating in exploitative systems.

When I brought up betrayal blindness with Stuart, he acknowledged that sometimes he probably avoids being fully aware of the injustice around him, just so he can keep showing up for his patients. Physicians I've talked with in every specialty can feel trapped for many of the reasons outlined previously — education debt, their spouse's job, needing to be near family or to avoid uprooting their children — so they put on blinders or make excuses for why their workplace is so dysfunctional. As a result, many of them are not entirely transparent with residents and students. They identify with the idealism of those young doctors and worry that talking openly about the realities of practice is needlessly discouraging at an already difficult time for trainees. Without that candor, residents may think they are the only ones struggling and that they need to find their own solutions, rather than adopting one of the various strategies modeled by their attendings.

Stuart loves teaching, seeing the energy and enthusiasm of young doctors who are ready to shake up primary care, much as he was ready to do thirty years ago. But by the end of their three years of training, they're unsure of their future. Every one of the residents Stuart has trained works half-time or less in clinical work, just like their mentor. Nearly 40 percent have gotten their MBA, planning an exit strategy from clinical work almost as soon as they've started it.

This exodus helps explain why the United States is facing an imminent shortage of physicians. The Association of American Medical Colleges predicts that by 2034, there will be nearly 130,000 fewer physicians than we need to care for our older and sicker population. In 2021, after two years of the COVID-19 pandemic, more than one in five physicians said they planned to leave clinical medicine within two years.[11] Many of those who do stay will reduce their hours so they can tolerate the distressing environment. Moral injury is at the heart of this despair.

CHAPTER FIVE

Mental Health Is Health

As Dr. Isabela Rodriguez walked into the emergency room for her first psychiatry consult of the day, the emergency room physician, Dr. Tim Ryan, waved her over. "Hey, Isabela, thanks for coming to see Xavien. She's in a tough spot." Isabela sat down at the computer next to Tim and started reading Xavien's record (in this chapter, names and details are anonymized). After a few moments, Tim rolled his chair closer to Isabela, who glanced over to him, expectantly. He cleared his throat, then said quietly, "Um, remember Danny — dark hair, big eyes, who painted his manic visions . . . ? He overdosed again last night." Tim paused. "This time the team couldn't save him."

Isabela knew Danny well. She had long dreaded having this conversation one day.

"Thanks for letting me know." Isabela felt tears welling up as she glanced at Tim, briefly meeting his eyes. *Buck up*, Isabela thought to herself, recalling what her grandfather, an immigrant from Cuba, told her whenever he saw her eyes glistening. But every day it was harder to do.

Composing her face, Isabela stood up from the computer. "I'll go see Xavien," she said.

"I'm sorry," Tim offered as she walked away. Isabela spun on her heel.

"I could have helped Danny, you know. But this godforsaken system wouldn't let me. He deserved better. They all do." Before Tim could respond, she turned and strode down the hall to meet the young woman who had just survived an overdose.

The rest of the day, between talking with patients, writing notes in the electronic medical record, and teaching residents, Isabela rehashed the many times she had treated Danny for his substance use and bipolar disorders. Though she was certain she had exhausted every possible avenue to get him treatment, the knowledge gave her no peace. By the end of the day, she was seething.

When her long list of consults was finally done, Isabela realized there was just enough daylight left to sneak in a ride. She grabbed her keys and raced from the hospital to the barn, where she saddled her horse, Beatriz, and charged into the wintry gloaming.

Tiny shards of sleet stung her face as she drove Beatriz hard uphill. The mare, who was bred for speed, was in peak condition after summer competitions. Flooded with adrenaline, Isabela hovered over the saddle, Beatriz's hindquarters lifting them airborne with each stride. The intense focus she needed to navigate around the hillocks and holes in the dwindling light momentarily pushed Danny from her mind.

When they finished the wide loop around the hillside, Isabela settled Beatriz and began the careful canter downhill. Just before reaching the bottom of the slope, she steered the mare toward a huge log they used as a cross-country jump. Today's ride was a conditioning workout, not jumping practice, so she hadn't prepared Beatriz's shoes with extra traction, but they both loved to fly and Isabela yearned for that boost today.

She felt the horse lock onto the obstacle and gather her powerful hind end under her. But two strides from the jump, Beatriz hit a patch of grass slick with frost and slid, scrambling to avoid crashing. Losing her balance, Isabela grabbed a handful of mane and just managed to stay atop her nimble mare.

"Ñoooooo! Comemierda!" she swore, pulling the horse to a stop. *I could have wrecked us both*, she thought. Her hands shook as she stroked the mare's steaming neck, as much to calm herself as to quiet the horse. Slumping forward, she burst into tears. As dark fell, Isabela sobbed for Danny and for every other patient with mental illness who suffered because her hospital and the mental health infrastructure in her state prevented her from helping them.

After a few minutes, Isabela gathered Beatriz, and they made the short trek to the barn at a walk. By the time Isabela unsaddled her horse, her face was dry. She ran her hands over the mare's legs, searching for the subtle heat of a new injury. Relieved to find none, she put the mare in her stall with a pile of fresh hay, then stood for a minute, listening to her chew, breathing in the sweet, earthy smell of the barn, before heading to the car.

During her three years at this hospital, the barn had been her sanctuary. Being with Beatriz was a way to escape her own pain, if only for an hour or two. But during the drive home, racked with guilt about their near miss, Isabela realized that if she had acted rashly here, her emotions might be getting the best of her elsewhere, too. She had been short-tempered with her boys at the bike park two nights ago and unwisely outspoken at a department meeting the day before. The frustration of working in a system that prevented her from helping her patients was coloring every part of her life and putting at risk what she'd work decades to build — her reputation as a skilled psychiatrist and a physician leader at her hospital and the patient, compassionate parent, partner, and horsewoman she expected herself to be. She desperately wanted something to change, but it wasn't likely to happen at her hospital, part of a large national, for-profit corporation, and having worked in two other jobs already, she knew the situation wasn't much different elsewhere. Just fifteen years into her career, Isabela was stuck: If she stayed, the work might break her, but she couldn't afford to quit.

Danny was only twenty-six when she met him, with doe eyes that made him look child-like and innocent. An artist, he painted jagged slashes of color on found pieces of wood or glass. He landed in the emergency room so frequently that someone on staff always recognized him; once he was coherent, he liked to show them pictures of his latest work. Opioid dependence, he told Isabela, felt like purgatory, because he didn't even get high anymore, he was using just to avoid withdrawal. For Danny, dope sickness felt like dying one frayed nerve ending at a time.

He grew up less than ten miles from where Isabela lives with her husband and two sons. Ten years ago, he was just a kid like her boys, messing around on his bike and playing video games. His father was the manager of a large supermarket and his mother was a receptionist in the business office of a local nursing home. They weren't wealthy, but they didn't want for much. Isabela wondered how Danny got hooked. Did he get Percocet for a sports injury, or from a friend at a party? She had learned that no matter your skin color, level of education, or the balance in your bank account, every mu receptor looked the same to an opioid. No one was safe from the scourge.

Isabela met Danny's parents once, just after she started working at this hospital, when they came in desperate to help their son. She found Danny a thirty-day inpatient program covered by their insurance, which got him clean. But getting clean and staying clean are two different things. Danny turned twenty-seven while he was in the hospital, aging out of his parents' insurance, so his outpatient care at a community mental health center wasn't covered. Ashamed to deplete his parents' meager savings, Danny decided to shoulder the costs himself, even though his job didn't pay much and he had no savings. Dwindling state funding and falling insurance reimbursements meant the treatment center couldn't afford to treat patients for free; if Danny didn't pay for his treatment on time, they would have to turn him away. Isabela knew Danny was set up to fail and, sure enough, unable to keep up with payments, he was turned away from treatment and relapsed within two weeks. His parents drained their savings to pay cash for a second thirty-day inpatient program. But without money for outpatient treatment, staying clean once again proved impossible.

Like many serious drug users, Danny always showed up in the emergency room alone after an overdose. When a friend found him unconscious, they would call 911, dose him with Narcan if they had it, then disappear as the ambulance arrived for fear of being arrested. The Narcan saved Danny's life, but in a flash, it locked up every opioid receptor in his brain, sending him into acute withdrawal. Worse than the physical effects — fever, vomiting, muscle pain — was how it ripped him from the womb-like comfort of his intoxication and tossed him into the wild anxiety of withdrawal. He would wake up spewing vitriol, throwing every ounce of his featherweight frame at the paramedics and the emergency room staff.

The emergency room nurses and doctors struggle to show empathy for patients like Danny who repeatedly overdose because efforts to save them seem futile. The opioid epidemic has been raging as long as most of the clinicians have been in healthcare, and yet hospitals, insurance companies, and policy makers refuse to allocate sufficient resources to fund effective long-term treatments. At Isabela's hospital, staff rescue overdose victims — they monitor vital signs, re-dose Narcan, refer to psychiatry, and absorb their post-resuscitation invective — but keep their emotional distance. Too many of them, at some point in their careers, grew hopeful about a patient's recovery only to pronounce them dead the following week.

Every day, Isabela had to remind herself these failures are not personal. She knew she was working in a broken system, but it was hard not to rage at the barriers to providing lifesaving treatments. As a psychiatrist, her emotions are her diagnostic tools, but to survive in her field Isabela learned to lock them away.

When she saw Danny after an overdose three months earlier, though, his arms and legs pocked with new needle marks, something about him cracked her armor. Danny was running out of veins and injecting heroin straight into his skin, which kept the dope sickness at bay a little longer but put him at risk for abscesses, flesh-eating bacteria, tetanus, and botulism. That night she didn't sleep for worrying about him, what his future would bring, and whether she could do anything about it.

Ideally, Isabela would have sent Danny to a five-day program to get him through the worst of withdrawal, followed by three weeks of intensive inpatient treatment. Then he would transition to a robust outpatient program that combined individual and group treatment with medication-assisted therapy for a minimum of two years. Dozens of studies have shown that comprehensive treatment programs save money for both hospitals and communities in the long run.[1] Yet most insurance companies and healthcare systems, whether they are for-profit or nonprofit, are obsessed with quarterly earnings and hesitate to make longer-term investments. Their performance is assessed in months, not years, and the shareholders and trustees are impatient to see returns.

If Danny were independently wealthy, he could wire payment to any one of dozens of private programs across the country and start treatment immediately. When he finished inpatient treatment, he could choose an outpatient program catering to his preferred approach to sobriety — yoga, rock climbing, art therapy, or something else. His best chance of success would be to stay in outpatient treatment for at least five years, at a total cost of $60,000 or more.

But Danny was indigent. He might be eligible for Medicaid, but he never finished the paperwork. Waiting lists were months long for the few publicly funded beds his region provided — just twenty beds for roughly eighteen thousand heroin users, most of whom were poor and uninsured. His next best option would have been a "bridge clinic" to help him manage the wait for a formal treatment program, but patients with substance use disorder are often unemployed and unin-sured, making it hard for those clinics to stay in business. Successful bridge programs receive taxpayer funding, either local, state, or federal money. But it is hard to convince taxpayers to support drug treatment programs when schools, roads and bridges, fire departments, and police officers also need those scarce dollars.

Isabela had no way to help Danny get clean, much less stay clean. All she could do after he overdosed was to call treatment programs in the hope of finding an open, publicly funded bed. When her search inevitably came up empty, before discharging him, she would implore him to follow up in the morning with a local free medication-assisted treatment clinic, where they would add him to a waiting list for inpatient treatment. Complicating matters, Danny used opioids to quiet the voices and visions he had when his bipolar disorder was out of control, but substance use disorder and mental health conditions were usually treated in different places, because of rules around funding. So like the 40 percent of substance use disorder patients with a dual diagnosis, Danny also needed to coordinate treatment at the local community mental health center. But long before any of the offices opened the next day, and because of the Narcan that saved his life, Danny would be dopesick and desperate for his next hit.

Watching Danny, like dozens of others, return to the same situation that repeatedly landed him in the ER felt to Isabela like betraying the oath she took when she became a doctor. She thought about quitting her job in protest. But she couldn't — she was the primary earner in her family and still had huge student loans from medical school. Besides, the hospital would just replace her with someone who would get stuck in the same cycle. Or worse, they wouldn't fill the position, leaving her patients without an advocate. Isabela went into the profession to help people heal, and she wasn't willing to turn her back on those who needed her. She just wanted the freedom to do her job.

In the fall of 2019, I met Isabela online through a group of women physicians who are also are devoted equestrians. We gravitated to each other as plain-spoken psychiatrists with similar approaches to support and shared frustrations about how medicine treats its workforce. During private conversations over Zoom, she related agonizing experiences in practice; sometimes telling the stories was so painful she would break eye contact or make jokes to escape the topic for a second. I could empathize; if I were still practicing, I would surely feel the anguish of moral injury as intensely as Isabela does.

Isabela grew up outside a large city on the East Coast. Her mother was a special education teacher whose family were among the first Europeans to settle in Virginia. Her father was the son of Cuban immigrants who fled during the Bay of Pigs invasion and was, like his own father, an engineer. Her maternal grandfather was a pediatrician and a psychiatrist, and her maternal great-grandfather was also a physician. The expectations for accomplishment ran deep on both sides of her family.

Encouraged by her Cuban grandfather, who had fond childhood memories of riding horses, Isabela begged her parents to let her take lessons at the barn down the street when she was in kindergarten. She relished the manual labor of caring for the horses — mucking stalls, stacking hay, hauling fifty-pound bags of grain, walking miles in pastures to find thrown shoes and unruly horses — which settled her fractious mind. Building trust with an animal ten times her size also helped her develop agency and leadership skills.

The grit, ferocity, and boundless energy that served her at the barn, coupled with a sharp intellect and high expectations, led to academic success all the way through college, when Isabela decided to follow her maternal grandfather into medicine. She got into her top-choice medical school but stumbled out of the gate and barely passed her first exams. The courses were harder than even her toughest classes as an undergraduate, and sheer intellectual ability no longer made up for poor study skills and wandering attention. Her adviser offered platitudes — she "wasn't alone" and "lots of students struggle, especially in the first year" — but Isabela didn't want to be just like everybody else, and she didn't want to struggle. Her goal was to be the best at what she did and to make it look easy.

Self-doubt crept in, and her confidence slipped in those first months. Then a friend told her about a pediatric intensive care doctor who spent half of his working hours flying to outlying hospitals in the medical helicopter to bring critically ill children to the academic hospital. Medical helicopters were known to be dangerous, and Isabela, an inveterate adrenaline junkie, was intrigued. When she tracked him down to learn more, they connected immediately. Isabela started spending some of her few free hours shadowing him in the pediatric intensive care unit, struck by his equally masterful ability to manage complex physiology and traumatized parents. Their time together helped her tolerate the brutal slog of classroom work, and by the end of her first year, becoming a pediatrician seemed within her grasp.

Then three weeks into her second year, Isabela's beloved adviser died when he lost control of his car on the highway and it rolled over, crushing him. In shock, Isabela felt unmoored, as if the promise he saw in her had died in that car, too. Over the next few months, she struggled to stay focused on her goals and her grades, barely passing her classes and her first set of licensing exams.

Isabela had always been aware that feeling physically unwell took a toll on her mental health and that the reverse was also true. Her grief for her mentor was not just deep sorrow; it was aching joints and heavy limbs. On her pediatrics rotation in the third year of medical school, she found herself constantly wondering how the child's psychosocial environment contributed to their illness. When her interest in mental health persisted during adult medicine rotations, she knew she had found her career path. She would practice psychiatry in the context of medical or surgical crises.

A few years before Isabela began her residency, workweeks were capped at eighty hours, so while the hours were still long, she felt rested enough to learn well. Her attendings were engaged, effective teachers who were committed to teaching residents the gold standard of psychiatric care. They also made time to teach residents about the history of mental health treatment and funding, particularly in the state where they worked. They wanted residents to understand why the system was so dysfunctional and to lay the groundwork for them to improve it.

In 1999, the Supreme Court handed down the *Olmstead* decision, declaring that mental health treatment must be delivered in the
least-restrictive environment possible, encouraging outpatient care
except in the direst circumstances, when the patient was at imminent
risk of harming themselves or others.[2] In response to the *Olmstead*
decision, Isabela's state passed legislation in 2001 that supported
privatization of mental health care. The goal was for the state to get
out of the business of directly providing mental health care to uninsured or publicly insured patients. Instead, they hoped to hand the
responsibility to private, specialized organizations that could work
more efficiently and with less bureaucracy. Then a budget crisis cut
funding in half, threatening the plan from the very start. During
implementation, leadership changed frequently at the Department of
Public Health, each time resulting in a new vision for mental health
care and a new management structure. The churn led to a disorganized, fragmented system. Services regularly disappeared as organizations went bankrupt or new leadership changed state plans. It was
confusing for patients and frustrating for clinicians.[3]

Staffing a clinic for low-income patients during residency, Isabela
saw what could happen on the rare occasions when funding and
opportunities lined up to provide comprehensive treatment. One of
her patients, Janelle, broke the cycle of her opioid addiction when she
was accepted for residential treatment off the waiting list. She stayed
at the rehabilitation facility for thirty days to get clean and to jump-
start her treatment, then was offered affordable housing and outpatient therapies as part of her recovery plan. Treatment, together with
the safety of a locking door, were the keys to her sobriety.

Isabela knew that Janelle had been lucky. Most low-income
patients would never have the opportunity to get clean — at the time,
her county had only ten beds for women who could not afford the
$10,000 per month price tag, either out-of-pocket or through insur-
ance coverage, for a treatment program. Even for those with good
insurance, the copays could be prohibitive. Even before she got out

into practice, Isabela began to feel like the deck was stacked against her, and against her patients.

At the end of her training, Isabela chose to take a job at the hospital where she trained. By staying, she could put her energy into learning to be an attending physician, rather than on relocating and adapting to a new organization; her husband also liked his job nearby and was reluctant to move. The trade-off was fighting to be seen as an attending where she'd done her residency, a notoriously difficult situation.

During her five years in that position, Isabela learned she preferred inpatient work and that she had a knack for psychopharmacology, but when she tried to do more of both where she was, she ran into roadblocks. The department wasn't divided into inpatient and outpatient work, and her burgeoning expertise with complex psychiatric management in the setting of a medical or surgical illness seemed to threaten some of the older physicians in her department. When she realized she had no clear path to advance in her career there, it was time to move on.

Isabela started looking for jobs where she would work only with patients in the hospital, whether admitted for medical or surgical care, or in the emergency room. After interviewing at two large academic centers, one nearby and one in the Mountain West, she got offers from both. With aging parents and elderly grandparents within driving distance, she chose the one across town. She was grateful she could change jobs without making a cross-country move, as many of her friends were forced to do.

At first, the new job was an improvement. Isabela felt supported by her administration and a tight-knit group of colleagues. But barely two months into this new job, her boss abruptly resigned, for personal and political reasons. Several beloved physicians departed with the chair, leaving the department reeling and understaffed, and Isabela stunned, wondering what was next. The pool of candidates who are leaders in academic psychiatry is small, and so many sudden vacancies suggested a department in turmoil, which might be challenging to lead. The search committee looked for a replacement for more than three years before finally hiring a new chair, who came in with big ideas about how to reshape the department.

Not long after the chair arrived, they declined to renew contracts for several of the long-term faculty who were not aligned with their vision. Isabela, who had been outspoken in the early months of the chair's tenure, debated whether to fight for a contract renewal when it came due the following year. Ultimately, she realized she did not want to pursue a career in academic medicine, with its myriad demands for clinical productivity, teaching, committee participation, and research. In late 2018, she started looking for a new job, this time for a position where she could focus on caring directly for patients and on training residents, a part of her work she had come to enjoy.

On the other side of her state, a large community hospital had established a psychiatry residency just the year before, and they were looking for a psychiatric hospitalist. It was the first vacancy in the department in five years because no one left the practice, except to retire. When Isabela interviewed, it was no secret that the century-old hospital was in talks with a for-profit corporation about a potential sale. The trustees were weary of worrying about the hospital's financial position; selling would allow them to endow a foundation with cash reserves that could see the community through a catastrophic crisis in healthcare. They even got the buyer to agree to build a new behavioral health center within five years, expanding inpatient capacity by 50 percent, to 120 beds. The chief medical officer, the chief operating officer, her department chair, and most of the faculty reassured her that nothing would change under new ownership. Satisfied, Isabela accepted their offer and moved with her husband and two school-aged boys to a new city for the first time in almost twenty years.

Shortly after she started work in the summer of 2019, the sale went through. Then nine months into her new job, the pandemic hit. Elective procedures shut down, and the hospital started hemor-rhaging revenue — a death knell in a for-profit system. Like at Fulton

County in chapter 2, where Hannah Becker worked, the administration took drastic action to control personnel costs, issuing new long-term contracts with steep pay cuts and a shift to productivity-based compensation. The actions sent shock waves through the organization.

Fifty-five doctors, or close to 7 percent of all physicians on staff, left to work elsewhere. Seventy percent of the psychiatrists left, so the five remaining psychiatrists, one of whom was Isabela, had to decide how to do the work of seventeen. The hospital scrambled to bring in locum tenens physicians to fill the psychiatry gaps, but a revolving door of temporary help failed to promote the same quality of care, or the same cooperation and collegiality within the department. Tempers frayed as consulting physicians waited, sometimes for days, for a psychiatrist to see their patients.

In early 2022, three years after the sale, the corporation was just starting to build the new behavioral health center that had been desperately needed during the pandemic when demand for mental health care surged. But it is likely to be some time before the hospital will be able to open the new beds even when they are finally finished. The corporation has earned a reputation among healthcare professionals for not treating staff well and has had trouble replacing staff who quit during the pandemic.

Because of nursing shortages, inpatient beds at Isabela's hospital are scarcer than they were before the pandemic. Every outpatient program has a waiting list, whether run by her hospital for insured patients or by community mental health centers for the indigent. The community intensive outpatient program for substance use disorder requires that patients who are in early sobriety show up for group therapy regularly, to show their commitment to treatment, before they are assigned to medication management or individual therapy. That's like saying to a diabetic, "You need to come to the doctor's office three times a week for two weeks to prove you really want treatment before we'll start you on medications or let you speak with a nutritionist." The barriers to treatment, even just the transportation costs of getting to appointments, for patients unlikely to have a job or healthcare insurance, are unnecessarily high. Patients like Danny are stuck on the street, without treatment, waiting to get pulled off a waiting list, and physicians like Isabela are helpless to do anything about it.

Talking with Isabela reminded me of my own experience struggling to provide mental health care in the face of enormous structural barriers. Mental health care is a uniquely challenging field; decisions about policies and payment systems are bound with attitudes toward addiction and mental illness and societal biases about who is deserving of care. Examining the roots of these systemic obstacles can help us understand why it has been so difficult to increase funding and improve treatment for mental health care.

In the late nineteenth century, the world was in the throes of the first opioid epidemic, and there were no meaningful international measures to control drug use and trade. Natural extracts like opium and morphine were pouring onto the world market from countries in Asia, and Bayer, a pharmaceutical company in Germany, had just extracted heroin, a drug they promised would relieve pain without risking addiction. Many patent medicines were laced with opiates and sold over the counter to the unsuspecting public. A 1905 exposé of the dangers of patent medicines by Samuel Hopkins Adams in *Collier's Weekly* motivated Congress to pass the Pure Food and Drug Act of 1906, establishing a precursor of today's Food and Drug Administration.

By the end of World War I, an international consensus supported regulation and containment, largely driven by fears about how narcotics could affect military readiness in the next great war. The Treaty of Versailles, which ended the war, contained Act 295, which constrained the manufacture, distribution, and use of addictive substances, with criminal penalties for violations.

Over the ensuing half century, public policy alternated between treating addiction as an illness and as a crime. Following the Pure

Food and Drug Act and Act 295, law enforcement cracked down on drug use and jails teemed with drug offenders. Henry Jacob Anslinger, head of the Bureau of Narcotics from 1929 to 1962, advocated harsh sentences for all habit-forming drugs, meted out by "tough judges not afraid to throw killer-pushers into prison and throw away the key."[4]

Other leaders took a more compassionate approach. President Calvin Coolidge tried to ease overcrowding in jails by signing the Narcotic Farm Act of 1929. Anyone convicted of a federal drug offense was sent to one of two narcotics farms run by the Public Health Service on huge tracts of land in Kentucky and Texas. Ordinary patients could also request treatment there. Each facility was an amalgamation of prison, voluntary treatment program, farm, and research center, and they quickly became famous for their country-club feel and their famous clientele, like musicians Sonny Rollins and Chet Baker and author William S. Burroughs.

Sadly, they also became infamous for their association with unethical experimentation. The Narcotic Farm Act also established the Addiction Research Center, whose groundbreaking experiments uncovered the previously unknown physiology and psychology of illicit drug effects, addiction response, and withdrawal. But a congressional hearing held by Senator Edward Kennedy in 1975 revealed the CIA secretly funneled money to the Addiction Research Center to investigate Russia's purported mind control drugs. Worse, researchers rewarded participants with the very drugs that landed them there, like LSD, heroin, cocaine, methadone, and cannabis. Both farms were shut down in 1976 and the facilities were turned over, ironically, to the Bureau of Prisons.

In the ensuing quarter century, public attitudes toward addiction became more sympathetic as better research revealed its biological underpinnings and psychiatrists changed how they categorized addictive behavior. In 1980, addiction was reclassified as a diagnosable mental disorder in the third Diagnostic and Statistical Manual. Previous versions of the DSM lumped addiction together with traits of sociopaths — exploitation, remorselessness, deceit, aggression, impulsivity, and lack of empathy. Though categorizing substance use as a psychiatric disorder marked a step forward, it was no guarantee of better access to treatment or more funding to support it, as mental health care had been systematically underfunded for decades.

Prior to the mid-nineteenth century, psychiatric patients were cared for at home, by family. As industrialization attracted more people to cities, family structure began to weaken, and many mentally ill people ended up homeless. Dorothea Dix, who believed humane treatment in beautiful settings would lead to cures, drummed up widespread support for using public funds to build asylums in each state to house and treat the mentally ill, following the fashion in Europe at the time.

For nearly a century, people with mental illnesses lived in asylums, separate from society, but treatment was hardly the bucolic vision of Ms. Dix. In 1946, Albert Maisel wrote a scathing expose in *Life* magazine of the appalling conditions in two psychiatric hospitals. Calls to close the asylums mounted, and by 1963, President John F. Kennedy, whose sister suffered a cognitive disability, signed the Mental Retardation Facilities and Community Mental Health Centers Construction Act, just weeks before his assassination. Community mental health centers would provide the outpatient treatment and support necessary for those with severe and persistent mental illness to reintegrate into their communities. The legislation provided seed funding for the construction of fifteen hundred centers and start-up costs for several years, after which they were expected to sustain themselves off insurance reimbursements.[5]

Unfortunately, the idealistic vision of community mental health centers broke down in the details of how to fund them for the long term, and fewer than half of the planned centers were ever built. Right away, it became clear that states underestimated how many patients were too ill to return to living in the community. When they tried to spread limited funds between old hospitals, which they needed to keep open longer than expected, and new community mental health centers, neither could operate effectively. They could not afford to treat patients for free, but too many patients were uninsured — even when they qualified for public insurance, getting through the paperwork was a challenge — and the centers struggled to make ends meet. Though many are still operational today, low insurance reimbursements and inadequate public funding to serve uninsured patients means community mental health centers serve a fraction of the patients in need of care, with a fraction of the services they would like to provide.

Even those with good private insurance often struggle to pay for mental health care, because most patients are responsible for a large portion of out-of-pocket costs. Until the Mental Health Parity Act of 1996, insurers could "carve out" mental health and substance use treatment benefits from medical and surgical benefits, meaning higher costs and fewer benefits for psychiatric illnesses, if they were covered at all.[6] As a result, reimbursement was so poor for inpatient psychiatric beds that most hospitals couldn't justify keeping them open. The Affordable Care Act in 2010 again tried to close the loopholes, but significant gaps remain. As Walter E. Barton, medical director for the American Psychiatric Association, wrote in a 1966 article, "service follows the dollar."[7] That is a truism for most endeavors, and it largely explains the dearth of mental health infrastructure today, but it can also be interpreted as an indictment of how our society chooses to invest in the health of our communities.

Clinicians like Isabela are left to wrangle with this imperfect system every day. One in five Americans are diagnosed with mental illness each year.[8] Fewer than half of US adults with mental illness, and just two in ten adults with substance use disorder, received treatment in 2020. Some don't seek treatment, but for many, finding care that is both affordable and available is so hard they give up and never get help.[9] Fewer than half of US counties have a psychiatrist, and insurance reimbursement is so low that 40 percent of them don't take insurance. One-third of counties do not have a psychologist, and two-thirds have no nurse prescribers trained in mental health.[10]

Dr. Will Torrey, the chair of psychiatry at Dartmouth Hitchcock Medical Center, a community mental health leader in New Hampshire for two decades, and one of my mentors, described the challenge in mental health care succinctly: "Discrimination against psychiatric illness has shaped our payment systems, but we need to realize that, sooner or later, psychiatric illness touches every one of us, in some way. The mental health business is everyone's business."

Isabela is a brilliant psychiatrist whose work ethic would make her grandfathers proud, but even when she's doing her very best, she is furious at the policies and payment systems that prevent her from being the doctor she wants to be. "I spent my twenties learning what constitutes the gold standard of psychiatric care," she told me during one conversation. "But the second I finished training and went into practice, I had to compromise because those gold standard treatments just aren't available, except to the independently wealthy. I know what my patients need. I know it's available somewhere, but I can't get it for the patients *I* see, in *this* emergency room, *today*, because our systems have made a choice that making a profit in healthcare is more important than caring for the community. That is really hard to live with."

Though she tries to keep her emotions on a tight leash, it would be only natural if her patients picked up on some of her distress. She takes her frustrations home with her and finds herself snapping at her husband and sons more than she would like. Even though her family knows her anger isn't with them, living with it is a challenge. Isabela knows it is only through hard work and plenty of forgiveness from her husband that the pressures of her job haven't ruined her marriage.

Physicians are some of the toughest, most resilient people I know, on par with many of the military personnel I met working for the army. That said, men and women sworn to care for others often struggle to prioritize caring for themselves. Like Isabela, many physicians have no choice except to figure out a way to tolerate moral injury indefinitely. Some blame themselves for not being clever enough to outsmart the system or self-medicate with alcohol, food, or shopping, for a temporary escape. A few dig in and fight back, crusading against the injustices they see. Many end up spent and just going through the motions.

As we will see in the next chapter, moral injury can have even more catastrophic consequences: Physicians die by suicide at nearly twice the rate of the general population.

CHAPTER SIX

Broken

In the summer of 2019, Dr. Elaine Pico sent me an email, asking if Simon and I could review a talk about physician distress that she planned to deliver at a national conference in the fall in honor of her dear friend and colleague Dr. Jacob Neufeld, who had died by suicide two years earlier. Dr. Neufeld, who went by Jay, was a specialist in pediatric rehabilitation and cared for children with severe disabilities, such as cerebral palsy, spinal cord injuries, and neuromuscular diseases. Garrulous and outgoing, Jay was a tireless advocate for the children in his care. He was also a humanitarian and a painter who used expired medical supplies as his tools. Elaine thought about Jay the moment she learned about moral injury, and she was sure it played a role in his death.

Three years before he died, St. Luke's Medical Center in Boise, Idaho, recruited Jay to set up a flagship pediatric rehabilitation program for the state of Idaho. But the month before Jay started work, the Federal Trade Commission filed an antitrust complaint against St. Luke's; two years later, St. Luke's lost the case and faced millions in penalties and lost revenue. In the wake of the judgment, money was tight, and as physician contracts came up for renewal, compensation changed from a fixed salary to a base salary with a productivity-based bonus. But in a specialty as complex as pediatric rehabilitation, seeing more patients in less time risked the very things that made Jay's program successful — thoughtful, comprehensive, collaborative care based on exhaustive communication with the patient and their parents. Putting those appointments on an assembly line set at an arbitrary speed was bound to lead to errors, complications, or worse.

Jay had been outspoken about the implications for patient safety when he learned of this shift. Then the surgeon who shared call with him abruptly departed, leaving Jay as the only doctor in the state who knew how to manage baclofen pumps, a notoriously fickle technology used by some of his patients. For six months, while he waited for administrators to replace his colleague, Jay was on call every minute of every day, because whether he was officially listed on the schedule or not, his colleagues would call him for help when they needed it.

I agreed to review Elaine's talk, and I asked if she would tell me more about her friend Jay. I wanted to understand how, in three short years, a dream job had become such a nightmare that a man full of life decided to take his own.

This is a story about one physician, told by the people who loved him, through the lens of their loss. I tried to get St. Luke's side of the story, but the administrators who interacted with Jay were unwilling or unavailable to speak. To learn about Jay and piece together the events leading up to his death, I spoke at length with Elaine and with Jay's wife, Wendy Neufeld; to his roommates in a treatment program in Mississippi; and to experts in physician health programs and medical board defense lawyers.

Everyone who knew Jay described him similarly, as an energetic, extroverted, Type A do-gooder who was, literally, an Eagle Scout. After college and in medical school, he organized charity events to support causes like hunger, homelessness, and AIDS prevention. In Idaho, his charitable activities supported the growing community of patients and their families at St. Luke's. He was known around the hospital for his colorful mismatched socks and rainbow shoelaces, which he wore to cheer up his patients. Jay even made house calls when he could, especially if his patients were nearing the end of their lives. After Jay died, Wendy met the mother of a former patient at a fundraiser, who remembered Jay bringing his small dog to visit her dying child. The mother told Wendy how the dog jumped up on the bed and tucked itself under the boy's arm while Jay sat beside them. All three stayed where they were until the boy passed. "I was upset until I saw my son was so happy. That was the best medicine Dr. Jay could have given him. He was the best doctor my son ever had," Wendy recalled the boy's mother saying.

Jay grew up in Moorestown, New Jersey, a suburb of Philadelphia. Though his own childhood was comfortable, the areas around Moorestown — especially Greater Philadelphia and New York — were ravaged by the collapse of manufacturing in the 1970s. When the tax base imploded, the funds both to clean the streets and patrol them evaporated. Muggings, gang fights, and drug deals were all over the evening news.

Witnessing those hardships shaped Jay. Even when Wendy met him in high school, he was street-smart and outspoken, especially on behalf of those with less privilege. After earning his degree in mathematics from Drew University, Jay returned to Moorestown while he decided what to do next. He joined the Rotary Club and within weeks convinced David Montgomery, owner of the Philadelphia Phillies, that the team should partner with his club on a combined food drive and fundraiser, "Strike Out Hunger." Still operating today, the program has fed thousands of families and raised millions to address hunger in local and international communities.

Jay wanted to do more about inequity than the occasional fundraiser, though. In 1986 he moved to Chapel Hill, North Carolina, to study for a master of public health degree at the University of North Carolina. There were a few young physicians in Jay's program, and through his friendships with them Jay became intrigued with medicine. As a physician, he could provide direct care and immediately relieve suffering, but he could also use research and advocacy to make change on a bigger scale. After attending Wake Forest University Medical School in nearby Winston-Salem, Jay moved to Detroit for his pediatrics residency and subsequent fellowships in pediatric rehabilitation and adult physical medicine and rehabilitation at Wayne

State University. Pediatric rehabilitation was an emerging field that promised to revolutionize the lives and care of severely disabled children. As clinical faculty at an academic hospital, he would be able to care for his patients while doing cutting-edge research. Jay couldn't imagine a better career.

After ten years of training, Jay earned a rare triple board certification — in pediatrics, pediatric rehabilitation, and adult physical medicine and rehabilitation — and began his first job on the clinical faculty at the Rusk Institute at New York University in 1998. Shortly after starting at NYU, Jay joined the university's disaster preparedness committee. For three years, he ran a busy clinical practice, serving on hospital committees, helping with regular disaster drills, and establishing his own body of research.

Then came September 11, 2001. NYU was the designated receiving hospital for any disasters in Manhattan below 14th Street, where the World Trade Center towers were located. Jay sprang into action to establish a center for families to get information about missing loved ones, and after just a few days, he was redeployed from his clinic to act as the liaison between the health system and the medical examiner's office, work he continued well into the fall.

When he returned to his regular duties, Jay found he missed the leadership role he took on during the crisis and decided to pursue a position with more responsibility. He began a pattern, common in academic medicine, of accepting a new position about every five years, ascending to increasing levels of leadership. In 2002, he accepted a position at the Medical College of Virginia as chief of pediatric rehabilitation. Just three years into his tenure, fellow physicians elected him president of the medical staff at the children's hospital. His reputation as a leader with vision spread and the Children's Hospital and Research Center in Oakland, California, a larger hospital with more research funding, recruited him to join their growing pediatric rehabilitation department. Jay was excited about the opportunity to work with a bigger team and to learn from his colleagues' diverse perspectives, so in 2006, he and Wendy moved again.

Just six months after arriving in Oakland, the director who recruited him left for another opportunity. Jay's colleagues knew he had leadership experience and encouraged him to step up to the position. After some days of consideration, he agreed to put his name up for consideration. Administration agreed, and he picked up where the director left off, training the team of specialists — nurses, social workers, physical therapists, occupational therapists, mental health specialists — to collaborate in a comprehensive pediatric rehabilitation program. In Jay's words, "Children's rehab is not just about the medicine; it's about how children live in the world. So, whether kids need help to eat better or get stronger or walk again, we're with them from beginning to end — in the hospital and clinic, at home and at school." He believed that making a big investment in children early on, across every dimension of their lives, would help them live more fulfilling lives as they grew up.

Oakland is also where Jay met Elaine Pico, a fellow pediatric rehabilitation specialist, who was on the same specialty recertification schedule — at the time, specialists had to sit for exams every ten years to maintain their certification. Jay and Elaine bonded over the shared pain of studying for those exams. They created a study group of colleagues across the country, which evolved into an informal support network in a niche field of medicine.

The study group often lamented the lack of a good journal for pediatric rehabilitation. Eventually, Jay decided to do something about it. With support from the Children's Hospital in Oakland, he founded the *Journal of Pediatric Rehabilitation Medicine* in 2009. Based on Jay's commitment to close collaboration with other disciplines, the journal required that every article have coauthors from different specialties. Yet again, it was just a few years before other systems came looking for him.

In 2012, St. Luke's Hospital and Children's Specialty Center began courting Jay to lead their pediatric rehabilitation program and to grow it into the preeminent center in Idaho. Jay was flattered, but he was savvy, too. Few doctors have enough training to treat the fragile patients with whom he worked. As he had in each of his previous positions, during contract negotiations Jay made sure St. Luke's had at least one other doctor on staff who could share call with him. He also secured support for his fledgling journal and a small amount of institutional funding for his research. Excited to take on a new challenge, Jay and Wendy left a community they loved in Northern California and moved to Boise in April 2013.

Jay had no idea about the turmoil he was walking into that spring. Beginning in 2009, St. Luke's embarked upon an ambitious expansion plan, acquiring twenty-two private practices in Boise and expanding its existing sites, including the children's hospital, by investing in programs like pediatric rehabilitation.

The buying spree ended abruptly after the purchase of the Saltzer Medical Group in December 2012. St. Alphonsus, the other big hospital in town, filed an antitrust complaint three months later, in March 2013, alleging that in buying the Saltzer group, St. Luke's created a near monopoly in the Nampa-Boise market. They asserted that as previous outpatient practices started billing as hospital sites, St. Luke's competitive advantage could drive up the cost of care by nearly 30 percent. When the Federal Trade Commission and the Idaho attorney general joined St. Alphonsus's complaint, the case became the first federal antitrust suit against a hospital system buying a physician practice.

The antitrust suit played out very publicly over Jay's first two years in Boise. St. Luke's lost the case in 2014 and lost again on appeal in 2015, and the judgment cost the health system more than $25 million — between forfeiting the $9 million investment in Saltzer, their own attorney fees, and the $8 million in attorney fees owed to St. Alphonsus.

Soon after the judgment, the executives who had crafted St. Luke's growth strategy — those who hired Jay and who had the vision for his program and the patience to let him build it — left the health system, either to retire or to pursue other opportunities. The children's hospital hired Dr. Kathryn Beattie, a pediatrician with an MBA from Columbia University, to be its new executive medical director. She had a reputation for improving finances, even if it meant straining her workforce.

Jay's program was subsidized by other departments because it generated a lot of downstream revenue from ordering imaging studies and laboratory tests and making referrals to other physician specialists, physical therapy, occupational therapy, speech therapy, and nutritionists. But especially in the wake of its legal and financial setbacks, St. Luke's wasn't satisfied with downstream revenue. Leadership also wanted more direct billing, which meant seeing more patients.

By 2015, Jay was under pressure to justify every minute of his day as billable time. On days he was at his clinic he started spending his lunch break dashing the half mile to the children's hospital so he could fit in one more consult. Whereas previously he had control over his schedule, so he could give his complex patients the time and attention they needed, schedulers now shortened his appointments and packed his clinics. When he overstayed his scheduled time with a patient, assistants would interrupt him and say, "Dr. Neufeld, your twenty minutes are up." Feeling like he was giving his patients short shrift ate at Jay.

In the fall of 2016, when Jay had been in Boise three and a half years, the physician who alternated call nights with him abruptly left St. Luke's for a job in another state. Until the hospital hired another physician who could manage baclofen pumps, Jay would be on call all day, every day, which meant he could never travel farther than a thirty-minute drive from the hospital. Because keeping him on call constantly for very long wasn't safe for him or his patients, Jay expected the hospital would start recruiting another physician right away.

As the days ran into weeks, and then months without a replacement, the constant call schedule took a toll on Jay. Like many physicians, he was edgy and slept poorly on call nights, even when the hospital didn't contact him. His requests for support from his administration grew more frequent and direct. Though he was proud of the program he had built, he started putting out feelers for other jobs.

At the same time, Jay's contract was up for renewal. In April 2017, after months of negotiations, St. Luke's presented a draft contract. Jay could live with the 30 percent cut to his salary, but the contract lacked provisions for call coverage, something Jay simply could not overlook. Wendy begged him to just sign the contract and get another job as soon as possible, but Jay refused. He told her that patient safety was a matter of personal integrity.

While his contract was still under discussion, Jay needed to be out of town for a weekend in May 2017. He had told his bosses months in advance, so they could arrange coverage for him, as was their contractual responsibility. They could have hired a temporary physician to work for the weekend, but they never did. Instead, the scheduler simply removed his name from the call schedule and did not identify a replacement.

With some trepidation, Jay left town on Friday morning. That afternoon, a child with a baclofen pump arrived in the emergency room in distress, maybe from a malfunctioning pump, maybe for some other reason. A baclofen pump is a small device, about the size of a can of tuna fish, tucked under the skin on the belly and connected to the spinal canal by a thin catheter snaked under the skin. The device delivers continuous, metered doses of a potent drug to counteract muscle spasms. A pump can improve quality of life for patients with conditions like spinal cord injuries, cerebral palsy, or multiple sclerosis — affording them the dignity of dressing and feeding themselves, for instance. But the pumps were prone to fail without warning. If the steady trickle of medication stopped flowing, the muscles could spasm unchecked. Overactive muscles can cause a rapid, uncontrolled rise in body temperature. As individual muscle fibers contract, they shorten and widen, compressing nearby capillaries and interrupting the inflow of nutrients and the outflow of waste materials. Muscle tissue in that situation may start dying in a matter of hours, leading to organ failure and even death.

The emergency room physician saw that no one was listed on the call schedule, but he was desperate and called Jay's mobile phone anyway. Jay spent hours on the phone, walking the physician through the workup. The child was admitted to the intensive care unit and their condition stabilized, but Jay was still worried. Knowing there was no one available to query the pump, he booked the first flight back to Boise on Sunday morning. When he landed, he went straight to the hospital to see the child for himself and talk with their parents. By Sunday afternoon, the child's condition had improved enough that they could be discharged. After six months of being on call, Jay's worst fears had almost come true.

St. Luke's had narrowly avoided a tragedy, and Jay hoped to leverage the crisis to wake up the health system to the consequences of its decisions. First thing Monday morning, Jay called Dr. Beattie to let her know he planned to request a review of the case. Given the stakes, he assumed she would support him, so he thought nothing of it when she asked him to meet in her office that afternoon. But the second he walked in and saw Dr. Beattie sitting next to her boss and a representative from human resources, he realized this meeting was not about the review. Jay immediately regretted not asking his lawyer to join the meeting.

Idaho is a one-party consent state, so before sitting down, Jay paused, as if answering a message, and texted his lawyer about what was happening, then called him, hoping he would pick up.[1] When his lawyer answered, Jay left the call live, put the phone in his pocket, and joined the meeting.

After he sat down, Jay later told Wendy, Dr. Beattie locked the door behind him. Then the human resources representative handed him the latest version of the contract, which he'd already refused to sign. They told him he had a choice: either sign it or agree to a psychiatric evaluation to assess whether he was an "impaired physician," a designation reserved for a doctor who is unable to fulfill professional or personal responsibilities because of psychiatric illness, alcoholism, or drug dependency.

Now Jay really wanted to speak with his lawyer. But when he asked if he could step out to make a phone call, the administrators told him they wanted his decision first, so he tried to quickly assess his options. He didn't know any other physician who had been through the evaluation process and frankly found the suggestion that he might be "impaired" baffling — he rarely drank, didn't do drugs, and wasn't demented — so provided his health insurance paid for it, Jay agreed to undergo the evaluation.

Two days later, Jay was on his way to Pine Grove, a treatment facility in Hattiesburg, Mississippi, well known to hospital administrators and state medical boards, for a psychiatric evaluation. Because Jay had nothing to hide, he was sure he'd be home by the weekend. Just like a patient who writes off the chest pressure of a heart attack as indigestion, his miscalculation would have dire consequences.

Medical board actions can be even more damaging to doctors' careers than malpractice suits. William Sullivan, MD, JD, a physician and attorney who represents doctors in medical board investigations, estimated that medical board disciplinary actions outnumber malpractice awards four to one.[2] And those actions have far-reaching consequences.

It is surprisingly easy to file a medical board complaint. It takes five minutes to fill out the online form, and anyone can do it, for any reason, whether mundane — a patient thought the doctor's office staff was rude — or egregious, like smelling of alcohol and slurring words during an appointment. The majority of complaints are baseless, and while some stop at the first medical board review, many are fully investigated.

Every investigation or disciplinary action by the medical board, hospitals, or professional societies must be reported to the National Practitioner Data Bank, a database operated by the US Department of Health and Human Services that contains medical malpractice payment and adverse action reports on healthcare professionals. The

National Practitioner Data Bank defines *investigation* so broadly that virtually any formal discussion of a physician's competence or conduct by any hospital committee must be reported. In Jay's case, St. Luke's almost certainly would have reported his impairment evaluation and suspension of hospital privileges pending its outcome. The board also requires colleagues to report any suspicion of mental or physical impairment in a fellow physician as a condition of their own medical licenses.

The National Practitioner Data Bank was established to protect patient safety, which it does very well, but there are few protections for physicians. Organizations like hospitals, nursing homes, and insurers can query the database anytime and usually revoke hospital privileges or remove physicians from payment panels if their license is on probation. If a physician cannot bill insurance, employers won't hire them, and even private practice can be a struggle since many patients balk at paying cash. Even more ensnaring, physicians who stop practicing for just a few years — if one's license status makes it impossible to get paid, for example — may be deemed unfit to return to medicine because their skills are out of date by the same medical board that made it impossible for them to keep up those skills.[3]

Ideally, physicians would avoid disciplinary actions. Each state has a physician health program set up, ostensibly, to provide impaired physicians with confidential, therapeutic alternatives to discipline. Physician health programs are separate from, but work in close collaboration with, state medical boards. In a case like Jay's, St. Luke's probably would have referred him to a physician health program called the Idaho Physician Recovery Network, which would coordinate with Pine Grove to arrange his evaluation and monitor his treatment. The collaboration is akin to a suspended sentence; as long as Jay went along with the plan, no official disciplinary actions would be taken. If Jay refused evaluation or, in Pine Grove's opinion, resisted any part of the program, however, Pine Grove would notify the Physician Recovery Network, which would report him to the medical board, and disciplinary action would follow.

Disruptive behavior on the healthcare team is exceptionally broadly defined; the Joint Commission, a body that certifies hospital safety and quality, defines it as "intimidating behavior that may compromise patient safety."[4] According to Gina Porto, RN, and Richard Lauve, MD, consultants who help hospitals address disruptive behavior, "Anything a clinician does that interferes with the orderly conduct of hospital business, from patient care to committee work, can be considered disruptive":[5] raising one's voice, not responding to calls, being cynical when discussing patient status, condescending language or tone, impatience with or reluctance to answer questions. While doctors and nurses are equally likely to display these disruptive behaviors, the power differential on healthcare teams and the resulting disproportionate effect of physician behaviors lead to physician interventions more often.[6]

Beginning in the early 2000s, healthcare systems grew concerned about the effects of stress and burnout on patient safety. Neither stress nor burnout is a formal diagnosis in the Diagnostic and Statistical Manual, the catalog of psychiatric disorders recognized by the medical community, but at the time, both were believed to increase medical errors, though the association was later refuted.[7] One frequently cited 2009 paper on the relationship between burnout and patient safety stated, "Substance abuse has long been acknowledged to cause physician impairment, which can result in disruptive behavior. Less well known is that stress, burnout, and depression, common psychiatric conditions, can result in similarly impaired patterns of professional conduct."[8] Although the intent of the paper was to encourage hospitals to protect patient safety by supporting these potentially impaired physicians, it had the unintended consequence of excessively broadening the "disruptive" label and opening it to potential abuse. Jay knew none of this when he agreed to go to Pine Grove.

Pine Grove, of course, wouldn't even confirm Jay had been a patient, because of privacy laws. But Wendy put me in touch with two of his roommates in the program, and with their help I pieced together what happened during his time at the facility.

The scope of Jay's initial evaluation at Pine Grove was very broad — from substance use to dementia to sexual habits. Jay's hair and urine samples were clean, neuropsychological testing showed no evidence of incipient dementia, and, as far as any of my sources knew, he was not anxious, depressed, or psychotic. Nevertheless, Pine Grove referred him to their Professional Enhancement Program for professionals with "interpersonal difficulties." Cal Goodrich, a pseudonym for one of Jay's roommates, said, "We used to joke, although it was not really a joke at all, that Pine Grove never met a physician they couldn't treat. Everyone who came for an evaluation ended up in one of their programs." Whether it was substance use, sexual addiction, trauma, or professionalism issues, Pine Grove had a program to treat it. Cal went on: "When I asked him why he was there, like we did with everyone, he said, 'I'm not really sure. They *say* I'm burned out.' He seemed sort of stunned by what had happened."

Both Cal and his other roommate, whom I'll call Jack Payne, described getting to know the same "Dr. Jay" that people in Boise loved. "Of all the doctors I've ever met or worked with — at Baylor, at Duke, anywhere — he was one of the top 1 percent," Jack told me. "He had a keen intellect, and his heart was absolutely in the right place. He was refreshing."

As part of the program, Jay, who had practiced yoga and meditation for years, led morning meditation groups in their apartment. He was stung when some of the participants laughed at him, refusing to take it seriously, but their reaction did not deter him from leading the sessions. He organized a large painting project, excited to share the joy and stress relief he had discovered in the activity several years before. And he purposefully miscalculated while grocery shopping, buying and preparing extra food so Cal, who was paying for the program out of pocket and consequently was tight on cash, had enough to eat. Just as he did with the children in his practice, Jay took care of Cal in a way that preserved his dignity.

In addition to meditation, the Professional Enhancement Program involved group and individual therapy, exercise, art projects, and Alcoholics Anonymous meetings, regardless of whether alcohol or other substances were a problem. The stated goal was to help physicians develop better interpersonal relationships, ethics, boundaries, effective communication, and work–life balance. Cal was troubled by the methods the program employed, though. "It was a confrontational style. You couldn't do anything right, and the staff would criticize you until you were broken. They assumed that all physicians were narcissists and obsessive compulsive and that the only way to 'fix' them was to break them down." In one case, Cal demurred from disclosing another participant's white lie, instead encouraging them to confess themselves. Cal was criticized for not informing on the other participant, rather than praised for helping the other participant find the courage to be honest with the group. Cal saw that dynamic repeated many times a day, in big ways and small. No decision was ever the right one. No disclosure was ever sufficiently truthful.

During the six weeks their programs overlapped, Cal watched Jay deteriorate. "Jay started questioning his sanity. He was much worse when I left than when he got there." Jack corroborated Cal's assessment and added that he felt Pine Grove had stripped away Jay's defenses and offered nothing as a replacement. "He went in confused and angry, and he was soulless after two months. He couldn't understand why giving his everything was not enough — why other people didn't value that."

Elaine Pico also worried about Jay. They had another board recertification coming up that fall, and she knew how conscientious and thorough Jay was about his exam preparation. The group usually started studying about six months before the exam, which that year was just after Jay went to Pine Grove. Technically, he was allowed to use his cell phone on nights and weekends, but the facility discouraged him from studying for boards or attending study groups, citing it as a distraction from his treatment. Elaine could hear how torn Jay was during her brief exchanges with him. If he studied, Pine Grove might claim he was noncompliant with recommendations, but if he didn't, he might not pass his recertification. Either way, he felt his career was teetering on the brink.

Participants in the program joked that no one left until their money ran out. Jay was initially enrolled in the Professional Enhancement Program for six weeks, but as he neared the end of his term, staff decided he wasn't ready to leave and extended his stay another four weeks. Cal was at Pine Grove for more than twelve weeks, and Jack, who had the best insurance, stayed for nearly six months. Prices are not listed on the website, but Cal estimated his costs were roughly $10,000 per week. Jack and Cal told me that many participants in their program paid out of pocket, for a variety of reasons — they'd been fired and lost their insurance, like Cal; burnout isn't a psychiatric diagnosis, and therefore insurance won't cover its treatment, especially in an intensive program; or insurance refused to cover any evaluation or treatment that is part of a disciplinary action. Facilities have business office personnel dedicated to collecting payment and identifying potential resources for participants. Jay's stay was covered by insurance, but he would still be responsible, as were all the participants, for five years of monitoring and treatment afterward, which might cost tens of thousands of dollars each year.

Ironically, while Jay was at Pine Grove at St. Luke's insistence, fighting to keep his license and his livelihood, the hospital replaced him with a young physician who had just completed fellowship. The young doctor was new to the workforce and likely didn't fully comprehend what it would mean to take solo call indefinitely. St. Luke's packed up Jay's office and had movers deliver the boxes to his house. He lost his program, his purpose, and the insurance that would cover the aftercare he needed to have any chance of keeping his license. For Jay, it was an enormous blow.

Wendy told me Jay came home "in terrible shape." He was with-drawn and despondent, overwhelmed at the prospect of another five years of this program as an outpatient. According to the Idaho Physician Recovery Network, "After successful completion of primary treatment, contract compliance includes total abstinence from addictive chemicals, continuing treatment, participation in physician groups, behavioral monitoring, random toxicology testing, work site monitoring, and attendance at Alcoholics or Narcotics Anonymous. Initially, therapy is weekly and urine testing is frequent." Jay had never felt like he belonged in the program, and now it would always hang over him. He was hopeless about his future in medicine and unsure how he would explain this experience to potential employers, when he didn't even understand it himself.

Although Pine Grove had no jurisdiction over Wendy, after she visited the facility for a family weekend, they recommended she attend therapy as part of Jay's post-release treatment plan. One day, just two weeks after he returned home, Jay was particularly distraught. Wendy was reluctant to leave him, but she was trapped — if she refused to attend even a single session, Jay's license could be on the line. Part of her wondered if she should refuse to go to the appointment and let Jay blame her for ending his career. At the same time, she worried he might never forgive her, so she went to her appointment.

While she was gone, Jay died by suicide.

The very first time I spoke with Wendy, she wondered if speaking up cost Jay his life. As mentioned in chapter 5, physicians have one of the highest rates of deaths by suicide of any profession. Most doctors don't get to that point, of course. Some quit, like Don Kovacs in chapter 3; some work less in clinic, like Stuart Pollack; and some suffer in silence, like Isabela Rodriguez. No matter how they respond, they are all victims of a profit-generating machine that has taken over healthcare.

One physician at a conference in December 2021 had the sobering experience of overhearing a conversation between non-clinician administrators, which they recounted in a private message.

> "I need them to produce. All the metrics are in place, and we need to increase profit. [The physicians have] had it easy. They've had their time and failed. Now we can take over and make this profitable for us," an administrator in his early 40s told his colleague. He explained how Olive Garden had reshaped its profit margins with subtle changes in the number of olives they added to each salad, then went on. "We need to find a way to have those doctors see more patients. If we can have them see 5 more daily, the revenue that can generate will be fucking fantastic for us. The customers can be our olives, but we want to increase our olives."
>
> "Customers? You mean patients, don't you?" His companion pushed back.
>
> "Same shit. Let's just call them PGUs [profit-generating units]."

Most administrators would not tolerate such crassness from their colleagues, but the concept of PGUs may be the ugliest caricature of an unspoken attitude inside many boardrooms of healthcare corporations. To quote an opinion piece by Dr. Danielle Ofri in the *New York Times* in 2019:

> By now, corporate medicine has milked just about all the "efficiency" it can out of the system. With mergers and streamlining, it has pushed the productivity numbers about as far as they can go. But one resource that seems endless — and free — is the professional ethic of medical staff members. This ethic holds the entire enterprise together. If doctors and

nurses clocked out when their paid hours were finished, the effect on patients would be calamitous. Doctors and nurses know this, which is why they don't shirk. The system knows it, too, and takes advantage. . . . In a factory, if 30 percent more items were suddenly dropped onto an assembly line, the process would grind to a halt. Imagine a plumber or a lawyer doing 30 percent more work without billing for it. But in health care there is a wondrous elasticity — you can keep adding work and magically it all somehow gets done. The nurse won't take a lunch break if the ward is short of staff members. The doctor will "squeeze in" the extra patients.[9]

But nothing is ever perfectly, infinitely elastic. There is always a breaking point. Some, like Jay, break physically or psychologically under the relentless assumption of "wonderful elasticity." Others survive only by breaking their oaths to provide the best care possible to their patients. Either way it is a tragedy for the profession of medicine and for the patients physicians serve.

CHAPTER SEVEN

Escaping Corporate Control

Deep in the first wave of the pandemic, a doctor I'll call Rita Gallardo posted a note on a private message board for physicians about having recently left her job at a local hospital to start a direct primary care practice (though her name is a pseudonym, the names of her employers have not been changed). She wanted to offer a lifeline to other physicians who might be feeling as trapped as she had just months before, when she realized her employer did not share her commitment to putting her patients first. Inspired by her courage, I contacted her and, after a brief phone call, decided that I would make a short detour on an upcoming road trip to meet her in person and talk in detail about her situation.

In late March 2021, during a lull between the third and fourth waves of the coronavirus pandemic, I drove from Carlisle to the small town three hours west of the Mississippi River where Rita lives, through lush Midwest grassland not yet parched by searing summer heat. Three hundred miles from the center of the contiguous United States, I was in the middle of the country, in every way. To reach Rita's farm, I turned off the dirt county highway at a big red mailbox that marked her lane and drove up a winding hillside flanked with trees. The sheltered lane gave way at the top to a sunny, gravel driveway bounded on three sides by the house and pasture fence. I parked under an ancient apple tree in full bloom, facing the unbounded area and one hundred acres of trails and hunting ground that spilled away behind the house.

As we walked around the farm, tending to Rita's turkeys, chickens, goats, and horses, her three young children chattered nonstop.

They'd grown unaccustomed to visitors during the pandemic and the novelty of a stranger was irresistible. So in fits and starts, between urgent requests from the kids, her story trickled out.

Rita was on active duty as a physician in the army during the early years of the War on Terror. She was deployed in the desert Middle East and witnessed the toll of combat in the shattered bodies of young service members. Confined to a military base ringed by Hesco barriers and razor wire, her only escape from those horrors was dreaming of the life she might build later, when she could put this all behind her. She imagined a husband equally enamored of country living, a sprawling farm where she could indulge her love of animals and her children could roam free, and a small-town medical practice caring for patients as she would care for her own family.

That dream sustained her through some awful days in the army. Later, when she returned to training to specialize in oncology, it was her touchstone. She met a man who shared her love of rural living, bought the farm I visited, and started the family they planned to raise there. But her professional life was far from idyllic. In the span of five years, she left two jobs when she felt pressured to practice in ways she felt were unethical, for the sake of a company's profit. Out of options for employment, she took an enormous risk and walked away from corporate medicine, striking out on her own and setting up a direct primary care practice.

At one point in our conversation, I told Rita that I admired her courage in forging a new path, to which she responded, "It's not all sunshine and roses — unless you count the thorns, too." She didn't have enough patients to support the practice yet, so she was away from home two to three weeks each month, doing temporary work to pay the mortgage on the farm and make payroll. "I don't know how long I can sustain both, and I don't know what I'll do if the day comes when I have to choose. I can't even think about it, so I just put my head down and keep going, one week at a time. Or sometimes just one day."

As I drove away, along the ribbons of dirt stretching through Midwest farmland, I thought about the sacrifices Rita has made to escape moral injury and couldn't help wondering what her horizon might hold.

Rita Gallardo spent her early childhood in suburban Southern California, surrounded by both sides of her extended Mexican–Native American family. Then in 1988, after her father's overleveraged business failed in the wake of 1987's Black Monday, her father moved the family to a small lumber mill town in the Pacific Northwest, where a friend had work for him. The town was hemmed in by national forests, and almost everything felt foreign to Rita. Her family went from being part of a community that looked like them and shared their culture to being one of the few minority households in the town. Rita was sure her parents had ruined her life.

Shortly after they moved, she and her father were walking down the sidewalk on one of the two main streets in town. A pickup truck slowed as it approached them and the driver shouted, "Injun!" as he passed. Perplexed, Rita looked to her father for his response. "What an idiot," her father replied, shaking his head. "He didn't even know enough to call us what we are." That moment of clarity, dignity, and sense of identity was powerful for Rita. Her father saw value in their difference and felt sorry for others who were not knowledgeable or curious enough to see it.

Rita took refuge from town tensions by riding ponies and studying hard. She excelled in high school and set her sights on a six-year combined college and medical school program in the Midwest. She could trim two years off the traditional path of four years of college followed by four of medical school, which suited her impatient nature. When she was accepted, she left the West Coast for good.

In her second year, she applied for a military scholarship for the medical school part of the program and was accepted. In return for free tuition and a stipend for living expenses, Rita would owe one year of active-duty military service for each year of education and training, but that seemed like a low-risk trade, given the United States had been at peace for nearly twenty years, with no major geopolitical conflicts on the horizon. She signed her contract for the scholarship and enlisted in the military in the summer of 1999.

Two years later, everything shifted in the matter of an hour.

On the morning of September 11, 2001, Rita was listening to the news on National Public Radio as she ironed her uniform before leaving for class when she heard that planes had hit the Twin Towers in New York City. An hour later, while watching the towers fall and the Pentagon burn on television, it hit her that her military service would look nothing like the peacetime engagement she imagined.

In 2004, Rita graduated from medical school and moved to a military medical base in the Southwest for her residency in internal medicine. During her first year of training, the insurgents in Iraq began using inexpensive improvised explosive devices (IEDs) to inflict dramatic injuries: Rolling over an IED triggered an explosion that turned an armored vehicle into an oven; soldiers patrolling on foot stepped on IEDs and lost both legs and the hand cradling their rifle. Only one service member suffered an amputation in 2002. The following year, 71 service members lost at least one major limb; in 2004 and again in 2005, about 150 lost limbs.[1] Ninety-two percent of service members wounded in Iraq or Afghanistan survived, compared with 75 percent in Vietnam, thanks to dramatic advances in military medicine and the heroic efforts of military medical teams.[2] Caring for severely wounded troops was an intensive undertaking, though, and the staff needed reinforcements.

Facing a shortage of doctors, Department of Defense leadership discussed whether to deploy trainees like Rita to fill the need. Ultimately, they didn't, deciding instead to extend deployments for military doctors and to call up more physicians from the Army Reserves, but the possibility of deployment sharpened the focus of every military resident and their mentors. The residents learned unconventional skills for internal medicine doctors — how to intubate someone with massive facial injuries, how to put in and manage chest tubes — in preparation for facing unconventional weaponry. They knew they would be going to war, and they trained, in medicine and leadership, for the lives that would depend on them.

Eager to test her readiness both to care for patients and to lead a medical team, Rita volunteered to deploy for a few months during her third and final year on a special clinical rotation in Landstuhl, Germany, the first stop out of Iraq or Afghanistan for wounded service members. For two months, she led the care of patients in the surgical intensive care unit, and by the end of that experience, she felt prepared to face her first duty assignment.

Throughout her medical education and training, like all doctors Rita was steeped in medicine's deep values. Simultaneously, she was immersed in the army's seven core values, taught in basic training and lived every day thereafter: loyalty, duty, respect, selfless service, honor, integrity, and personal courage.[3] A shared commitment to these values forged impenetrable bonds among service members. Each individual was ready to sacrifice themselves at any moment, for another or for the group, without question. Almost every military physician saw evidence of that sacrifice every day, drawn on the bodies of young service members who followed orders into harm's way. It was a constant reminder of the honor and hardship of living an oath.

Rita's entire military service was during wartime. Immediately after finishing her residency, she deployed to a noncombat post where she was the only doctor for a battalion of a thousand service members. Despite her junior rank, combat leadership looked to her for guidance. When she rendered a medical opinion about a question or a concern they raised, no one googled the information or sought a second opinion. They incorporated her recommendations into tactical considerations and moved ahead. After a year at that duty station, she returned home for a short break, then deployed again, as a battalion doctor in the Middle East. There she was promoted to brigade doctor, responsible for the care of six thousand service members. In this role, she briefed senior officers, equivalent to the CEO of a company, and defended her decisions to them with data, objectives, financial impact, and rationale. Along the way those typically brusque leaders mentored, educated, evaluated, and groomed her to take on increasing levels of responsibility.

Rita's maturation as a military officer and a physician leader is the result of a painful lesson learned by the military during the Vietnam War. In March 1969, US troops killed at least 175 noncombatants in My Lai. When the event and its yearlong cover-up were revealed by investigative journalist Seymour Hersh, General William Westmoreland called for an investigation of army culture and professionalism, which was conducted by the US Army War College in 1970.[4] The resulting study identified many of the features of eroded professionalism and dysfunctional self-interest that permeated the army, including an "overemphasis on measurable results (a prominent feature of bureaucracies) such as body counts, training activities, and maintenance statistics; inadequate training; careerism; and many other indicators of, in particular, an Army officer corps often more interested in individual advancement than in mission effectiveness and soldier well-being."[5]

A follow-up study in 2000 found recurrent tension between the bureaucracy necessary to run a huge organization like the army and the professionalism of those who work under the control of that bureaucracy. In response, the army recommitted to developing the professionalism of its members, through policy, doctrine, training, and education. It even created a Center for the Army Profession and Ethic at West Point.[6] Rita's professional development was shaped by those reports, and by the recognition that while bureaucracy is a necessary part of large organizations, it must not subsume the profession it supports. Developing each of the four pillars of professionalism — technical skills, human development, professional ethics, and culture — primed Rita to recognize conflicts between the bureaucracy of large healthcare organizations and the profession of medicine.

A career in the military had never been Rita's goal, so while she would always be proud of and grateful for her service, she separated from the army when she was eligible. After seven years of active duty, she was ready to pursue her true passion, cancer care, and was excited to return to her medical school's hospital for her three-year hematology-oncology fellowship.

Shortly after beginning her fellowship, Rita committed to two partnerships. The first was with her future husband, Rudy, whom she met two months into fellowship. The second was with Tanner, a fancy young horse she imported from Europe and whom she planned to train herself. During her fellowship, Rita and Rudy married, and when she finished, they decided to settle in his rural hometown, ninety minutes from any major city, where they would be surrounded by his extended family and close to many of Rita's colleagues from her fellowship. She was ready to put two more huge pieces of her dream into place — buying land for her family and caring for her community as the doctor she always imagined she'd be.

Rita arrived in her husband's hometown in the mid-2010s, eager to put down roots and full of idealism about what she could bring to the fifty-bed local hospital she joined, where she would be the first oncologist on staff full-time. Before taking the job, Rita spent months painting a picture for the administrators of the comprehensive oncology care clinic she envisioned, with nurses to give infusions, a specialty pharmacist, and a social worker dedicated to helping patients manage the psychosocial and financial aspects of their diagnosis. Rita would be able see patients as soon as their primary care physician first worried about cancer and expedite the evaluation, rather than waiting to see them until after their diagnosis was confirmed. Plus, her patients could access chemotherapy infusions close to home, rather than driving two hours to the nearest clinic. She thought patients and primary care doctors alike would be grateful for access to a full-time oncologist, rather than one who was in town just a couple of days each month.

During those conversations, the administrators seemed excited about her vision for oncology care, but once she arrived, something seemed off. Rita thought their enthusiasm meant they agreed with her and would willingly provide the necessary resources for her to start the clinic. She didn't realize that sometimes in corporate culture, feigned enthusiasm is nothing more than a conflict-avoidance stall tactic, like a weary mother's "maybe." Before long, she realized her leadership hired her, as they did all physicians, to generate revenue; they hired administrators to strategize and to lead. If she wanted to build something bigger, she would first have to prove she could bill her worth.

After months of lobbying, the administration let her set up her clinic in one of the defunct inpatient hallways, with two nurses assigned to administer infusions. Two years later, the clinic was so popular it needed more space. It was also very profitable, so it took little convincing for the hospital to build a new clinic, designed to Rita's specifications, with two hallways of exam rooms, a break room for the staff, and infusion rooms that looked like hotel suites.

Just after her fourth work anniversary, the new clinic opened with a full complement of staff: half a dozen nurses giving infusions, a specialty pharmacist, and a social worker. Her vision of creating a cancer clinic in the local community, so patients could get big-city care without the drive, was thriving. But her relationship with the hospital was fraying. Rita started to realize she had irreconcilable differences with leadership the day she came out of an exam room and found the physician who was her electronic medical record coach waiting for her.

"Hi, Rita," Larry began. "You know Cindy, the practice manager — she asked me to see if I could show you a few tricks to be more efficient."

Rita met his smile with an impassive stare.

"Mind if I take a look at your notes? Mr. Galea, right? Oh . . . his chart is empty. Maybe you were seeing someone else?"

"No, you had it right. I was seeing Mr. Galea."

"Oh, well then. Let me show you a few things," Larry said, eagerly diving into a demonstration of EMR shortcuts and templates for her notes and orders. Rita stopped him mid-keystroke.

"I know the keystrokes for those shortcuts. That's not why I took a long time," she explained, meeting his gaze. "I *chose* not to use the EMR while I was in the room with Mr. Galea because his cancer is now incurable. He'd already sensed that was the case, but his wife of forty-five years was having a hard time processing the information. She was sobbing and needed some support after hearing such devastating news. So thank you, but I think I understand all I need to know about the EMR and efficiency."

Leaving work that day, Rita realized her conflict with the hospital was bigger than the EMR. Her employer's very goals were at odds with compassionate care.

The final straw came just a few months later when the hospital leadership negotiated a deal with a large healthcare system to take over the clinic Rita had built. "I thought, like in the army, I was in the lead. If I saw a need, it was my obligation to create something for the community. But within a few years, through a series of corporate transactions that didn't include me, the system showed it was happy to make money with my ideas and my sweat equity, but it wasn't going to give me any credit for my organizational abilities. Instead of thinking 'What an asset,' my administrators thought I was in their way." Despite earning more than she ever had in her life, Rita had never been more miserable. She couldn't do the job she loved, and there would never be enough money to make up for that. "I was in a very dark place, and I didn't see any way out." For months, she cried every day after she put her children to bed, wondering why she couldn't just compromise, if only for their sakes. Was there any way she could still practice medicine with integrity?

Rita fantasized about running her own private practice, where she could control every aspect of patient care. But none of the doctors she knew ran their own practices; she wouldn't even know how to start. Like Don Kovacs in chapter 3, her mentors in primary care had all sold out to hospitals or healthcare systems and become employees or retired and shuttered their clinics. Then in December 2019, she noticed

on social media that her fellow army scholarship colleague from medical school had opened a private practice. Rita immediately got on the
phone and during her forty-five-minute drive home, listened to her
friend explain the "direct primary care model" she was using. "It's the
same thing we were doing in the army — setting up and running a
clinic. You'd have no problem," she reassured Rita. By the end of the
phone call, Rita was convinced she could open her own practice, too.

Direct primary care practices are small practices that allow for
personalized care and direct access to the physician. Doctors typically
care for six hundred to seven hundred patients, instead of the two
thousand in a typical primary care practice, so appointments are long,
and they can spend as much time as they need with each patient. Such
practices typically do not accept insurance, instead charging patients
a monthly fee, usually around $50, and maintain very low overhead so
as to pass savings directly to patients. Most direct primary care practices negotiate special cash rates for testing and imaging, which, like
the monthly fee, are a fraction of typical charges — $400 for an MRI
rather than $2,000, for example.

During her few days off over the year-end holidays, Rita pored over
state laws about running a clinic and medical licensure, scoped out
office space, and drew up a rudimentary business plan. In late January
2020, she filed paperwork to establish her business. Finally, she turned
in her resignation and negotiated a new position at the hospital across
town, so she would have another source of income if and when she
launched her direct primary care practice. Her new administrators
allowed her to insert a clause in her contract that she would be able
to work at her own clinic in addition to her duties at the hospital.
For Rita's part, she preferred the stability of an employed position to
the uncertainty of entrepreneurship, and she wanted to believe there
might still be a place for her inside a health system. It took only a few
months to disabuse her of that fantasy.

Mrs. Alvarez came into Rita's oncology clinic late in the summer of
2020, tired, bruised, and aching, after a lab test ordered by her primary

care doctor showed some abnormal blood cells. A thorough workup pointed to a rare blood cancer, one Rita had seen only once before, and the prospect of treating it made her uneasy. Her instinct was to send Mrs. Alvarez to a more specialized center, which happened to be part of another health system, because all the doctors in her system were similarly unfamiliar with this rare blood cancer. But her new hospital regularly reminded doctors that they were expected to refer within their own system. Though it was illegal to threaten physicians directly, Rita knew her administrators were tracking her referrals, and they hinted at serious consequences if she failed to comply with their expectations.

Rita knew the perfect person to see her patient: her mentor from her oncology fellowship, an expert in rare blood cancers who had treated hundreds of similar cases and worked at the academic center just seventy-five miles away. He was also a gentle, kind man who would take the time to make sure Mrs. Alvarez understood what he was doing and why. Rita made the referral wondering what the repercussions would be and how long it would take anyone to notice.

Just a few weeks later, she got her answer. At her quarterly performance review, in early October, the administrator who was her supervisor reviewed her patient satisfaction scores (excellent), her outcomes (good), and her productivity measures (could be better). Then he raised the topic that seemed to be his sole focus these days.

"Dr. Gallardo, I'm concerned about your pattern of referrals. You've sent more patients outside the network than any of our other oncologists."

"I only do what I believe is best for my patients. If what they need is available in our system, then that's where I refer them — and you'll see I've done that plenty of times. But if we don't offer what they need, I'll send them where I think is best."

"Can we talk about how to do better?"

Rita squared her shoulders and took a slow breath. She'd been through this before and knew that losing her temper would only hurt her case. In a measured tone, she responded, "I'm doing the very best

I can with what we have, but I am not interested in any tips about changes that wouldn't help my patients and would only help your bottom line. Now, if you'll excuse me, I don't want to keep patients waiting. That really does a number on my satisfaction scores."

The administrator stared, his jaw slack, as Rita stood up and left the room. Walking down the hall and around the corner, she stepped out the back door and a blast of steamy late-summer air took her right back to the desert, where she had been the expert. There, the strength of the fighting force was at risk and her word had been law. She would have given almost anything to have a fraction of that autonomy now.

She took a few long, deep breaths and ran through her limited options. To keep this job, she would have to comply with the administration's expectations about productivity and referrals, but doing so would require surrendering her integrity. She already felt rushed through very difficult conversations about life-changing diagnoses. Cutting appointments shorter felt cold. Referring patients to doctors who weren't a good match for their conditions, to keep revenue in the system, felt downright wrong. How could she make those referrals and still tell her patients she cared about them and had their best interests at heart?

Rita knew the warning signs of a healthcare system whose goals conflicted with her own and how awful it felt to try to stay in a situation like that. But she had carefully evaluated each of the local healthcare systems just nine months before, and none of the other hospitals in the region was a viable option. It might be years before she could support her family on the income from a direct primary care practice. If she left this job, she would have to move her family or live away from them to work for another healthcare system. She was starting to fear that she would soon have to choose between caring for her family and caring for her community.

There were a lot of things about how Rita's employers wanted her to work that she found objectionable, but the one she just couldn't get past was the push to keep revenue within the system, at almost any cost. In the military, Rita had been sheltered from the business of medicine. As she started learning how and why money flowed in corporate healthcare, she began to understand why she felt so trapped.

Since the late 1980s, hospital corporations and healthcare systems have been exerting ever more control over how doctors practice. Healthcare systems use various explanations for why they need so much control — to standardize operations across a huge corporation in the case of Hannah Becker in chapter 2; to improve care measures in the case of Stuart Pollack in chapter 4 — but the common denominator is money. When Rita referred patients to doctors working in other health systems, she was creating what is known in the business language of healthcare as referral leakage, which in turn causes revenue leakage, and it is as ugly and as messy as it sounds.

Typically, referrals beget more referrals as specialists try to reach a definitive diagnosis, or to treat a condition. In 2014, a business management company looked at orthopedic surgeon referrals from primary care doctors — because musculoskeletal complaints are common, orthopedics referrals are also common. Thirty-seven referrals to an orthopedist led to seventy-four office visits for initial evaluation and follow-up; fifty-nine in-office diagnostics, such as an X-ray; twelve in-office procedures, like steroid injections; thirteen surgeries; and seven referrals to other clinicians, such as physical therapists.[7] Each of those incidents of care generates revenue, so the more that stay in the system, the better for the bottom line.

In 2018, a referral management company commissioned a survey of 104 healthcare executives about patient leakage. Eighty-seven percent of the executives said reducing patient leakage was a top priority and one in five admitted the phenomenon was draining more than 20 percent of their projected revenue.[8] Every appointment made outside the system represented, on average, $210 the organization did not earn. With estimates of a hundred million specialist referrals every year, such "leakage" quickly adds up to billions of dollars.[9]

When healthcare systems nudge patients to get care in a particular place or from certain clinicians, it's known as corporate steering. Because direct incentives are illegal, organizations use a variety of other tactics to steer referrals where they want them to go, such as strongly worded reminders to physicians about how internal referrals improve continuity of care, communication, tracking to ensure follow-up, and patient satisfaction. Most health systems also employ referral coordinators, who typically send patients to clinicians or testing sites within the healthcare system, because they don't have relationships with clinicians elsewhere.[10] Automated referral programs default to in-system entities, without giving patients a choice of location or clinician, and order templates for labs or radiology studies are emblazoned with the name of the healthcare system and the addresses of in-system locations. Many patients believe that those locations are the only places where the orders are honored when, in fact, they can fill them anywhere.

Several studies have looked at how ownership influences referral patterns. One 2018 study found that employed primary care physicians in Massachusetts are almost twice as likely to refer patients to a specialist within the system that owns their primary care practice as to specialists outside their system.[11] In 2019, a PhD student looked at referral patterns before a practice was bought by a larger healthcare system, and what happened after the acquisition. Medicare data showed that physicians whose practices had been bought by a hospital referred patients to that hospital nine times more often than they had previously, an increase driven by a commensurate drop in referrals to independent clinicians. When hospitals sell practices, the opposite happens.[12]

Administrators, keen to change stubborn habits, closely track physician referral patterns by extracting data from the EMR or from insurance claims. If that data identifies a physician as making too many outside referrals, a physician leader (like the chief medical officer), an administrator, or a dedicated "physician relations team" (whose job it is to manage physician behavior) has a conversation with the physician and reminds them of the implications to the bottom line of referrals outside the system.[13] Of course, doctors like Rita Gallardo hear the unspoken message that these decisions could affect their job security.

The pressure on physicians to refer in-house can also come from insurers. When a physician refers outside of their health system, that other clinician may be "out-of-network," which can incur significant additional costs for the patient and the insurer (who may not have favorable rates with the outside clinician or facility). That can make for unhappy patients, whose care is more costly than they expected, and unhappy insurers, who must pay higher costs for care.[14] Many patients have learned to ask whether a specialist they have been referred to is "in-network," rather than asking if they're the best fit for their condition.

Government agencies, healthcare corporations, and consultants often insist that keeping care in a single system means better outcomes for patients. To date those claims haven't held up to scrutiny. One study of cardiologists in 2018, for example, found that more consolidation of practices led to increased mortality for their patients.[15] Another study that same year found no improvement in quality of care at hospitals that acquired physician practices compared with those that did not.[16] It would be hard, then, to fault doctors who want to continue their previous practices of matching patients with experts they personally know, whose quality of care they trust, or whose interpersonal style would suit a patient well.[17]

Healthcare systems have gone to a lot of trouble to create workflows and constant reminders that make it easiest to refer patients within their own network. But the path of least resistance isn't always the way to the best care.

Rita had never been one to do what was easiest. As she always did when faced with a difficult decision under duress, she leaned on the army values that had served her so well — duty, honor, integrity, and personal courage.

On the drive home that October day, she thought about the community she had come to call home. So many people, too many of them living in poverty, needed better access to high-quality primary care. She and Rudy had moved to this town to be near family, and she did not want to uproot her children. By the time she pulled into her parking spot beside the ancient apple tree still adorned with the last remnants of the fall harvest, she'd made her decision. As her children raced across the grass to greet her, she knew the only way to keep this life and stay true to herself was to go all-in on the direct primary care practice.

She paid cash for a foreclosed 1940s building in a tiny town just down the state highway from her farm. The house is next door to a gas station and general store, halfway between the high school and the United Methodist church. There are hospitals in each cardinal direction from her new office — fifteen minutes north or south, double that distance east and west. For the first few months, Rita, Rudy, and members of the community worked nights, weekends, and holidays to turn the building into a medical office: installing ramps, rails, a locked medication room, a new refrigerator; giving it a fresh coat of paint. She bought barely used equipment at bargain prices from one of the local hospitals that was redecorating and furnished the waiting room with donations and thrift store purchases.

The practice is both bare-bones and full-service. Rita employs only herself, a part-time nurse, and a part-time receptionist. She sees her patients in two-hour-long annual appointments and hour-long follow-ups, though she will take as long as a patient needs and will even make house calls if mobility is an issue for someone. She contracts directly with laboratories and imaging centers so her fees for tests are a fraction of those at the local medical center, often less than a typical insurance copay.

Direct primary care isn't a panacea, though. Rita is on call all day, every day, all year long. If she had been saddled with education debt, she might not have been able to choose this path. Like most physician families where both partners work full-time, Rita and Rudy have a team of people helping at home — Rudy's extended family and a live-in nanny — otherwise, such a schedule would be impossible with three young children. Her panel of patients is much smaller than a traditional physician practice, which allows her to spend the extra time with each person, but if all primary care doctors changed to the model, it would be hard for patients to find a doctor. Rita doesn't participate with insurance companies, so patients must be able to pay her fees, as well as insurance premiums for a high-deductible plan or health savings account in case of emergencies. And it's not a model suited to many specialists whose care is episodic (not many people need regular care from a cardiothoracic surgeon, for example) or who require sophisticated technology or specialized facilities, like operating rooms.

Rita's office has tiny slices of her personal life scattered about — a picture of her beloved horse on one exam room wall, and on another, a steel plaque, made by a patient, that reads DON'T CALL IT A DREAM, CALL IT A PLAN. She doesn't miss her fancy office, a big staff, or all the latest diagnostic equipment. Those things were meaningless when she struggled to get her patients the care they deserved, with the specialists she thought were best for their situation. But she's paid a high personal cost for this freedom. Less than a year after I visited the farm of Rita's desert dreams, she and Rudy decided to sell it. The uncertainty of direct primary care income, especially in the early years, meant that many months they found themselves scrambling to pay the mortgage. They downsized to a smaller farm with one-tenth the land and hope that sometime in the future they can revisit the bigger dream.

Rita found a sliver of hope in direct primary care. It's too soon to know whether she can really declare victory, but for now, she's healing from her moral injury by healing her community according to the values she's long lived by.

CHAPTER EIGHT

Communities Destroyed

On Thursday, December 9, 2021, Dr. Priya Mammen hustled her kids out the door to catch the school bus, then sat down with one more coffee while she browsed the *Philadelphia Inquirer*. The regional news about the business of healthcare seemed more tumultuous every day. BRANDYWINE AND JENNERSVILLE HOSPITALS WILL CLOSE, LEAVING THOUSANDS IN CHESTER COUNTY WITHOUT NEARBY EMERGENCY CARE, read the headline.[1]

While she was skimming the piece, her phone chirped with a text from a nurse she'd become friends with when they worked together in the Jennersville Hospital emergency room. "That eerie sound we've been hearing in the background? It was Tower Health circling the drain." Just three years earlier, Tower Health had purchased Jennersville and four other small hospitals in the region in a bold bid to challenge encroachment from other large healthcare systems.

This news had been a long time coming, but Priya was surprised how frustrated, disillusioned, and sad she felt when she thought about how losing the hospital would affect the community around West Grove, Pennsylvania. Some of her patients at Jennersville — a diverse mix of farmers, horse breeders, factory workers, Amish families, professionals, and urban transplants — were among the sickest she had ever treated. Most of the farm and factory workers were uninsured or underinsured and earned hourly wages; they had little paid time off and couldn't afford to miss work, so they waited to get care until their bodies gave out. Frail elderly residents of a local retirement community also depended on the Jennersville emergency room; the next closest hospital was twenty-two miles away, a thirty-minute drive that would feel like an eternity in a life-threatening emergency. Closing Jennersville would also mean shutting down Medic 94, an ambulance service run by the hospital that handled most transfers out of the county.

Priya had liked her job at Jennersville, where she worked for nearly two years, from May 2019 to March 2021. Her hour-long commute took her through rolling fields to a place that felt like home, twenty miles down Route 48 from where she grew up in Greenville, Delaware. Then the pandemic hit, and Jennersville, like Fulton County Medical Center in chapter 2, started bleeding revenue. By the fall of 2020, Tower Health was trying to sell off the five smaller hospitals and twenty-three urgent care offices in its network but could not find a buyer. When Jennersville let Priya go a year into the pandemic, in the second of three rounds of layoffs, it was both a personal blow and an ominous signal about the future of healthcare in the Greater Philadelphia region. The city had lost ten thousand healthcare jobs between February 2020 and February 2021,[2] and with more cuts on the horizon, Priya worried for her patients, who would have fewer options for care, and for her colleagues, who had few opportunities for work in the area.

In the fall of 2021, Tower Health announced it had found a buyer for two of its hospitals, Jennersville and Brandywine, and the community breathed a collective sigh of relief. Now, mere weeks before the sale was slated to happen, Tower canceled the deal and announced it would close both hospitals. It was over for Jennersville.

Staring out her kitchen window, Priya thought about how the hospital's closure would reverberate through West Grove and the Greater Philadelphia community, abandoned by the healthcare corporation that had pledged to care for them. It was an unmistakable echo of her own betrayal by the profession of medicine.

Before she was born, Priya's parents, who are both doctors, immigrated from India to Wilmington, Delaware. Physicians who train in other countries still need to complete residencies in the United States to qualify for a medical license, so Priya's father, who was already a general surgeon in India, repeated his residency in surgery after they arrived. Her mother, who left India partway through her obstetrics training, opted to retrain in psychiatry, knowing a more predictable schedule would make it easier to care for her family without the support of grandparents nearby.

Priya grew up surrounded by family and friends who were physicians. It was a joke in her house that no holiday gathering was complete without at least one of her parents, and sometimes several guests, excusing themselves to attend to a patient. Her parents talked with Priya and her younger brother about the promise they had made to their patients, so Priya accepted their absences as normal, not knowing any different until she was older.

Despite plenty of positive role models, Priya wasn't interested in becoming a doctor herself when she went to college. While she was exploring majors in her first year at Tufts University, she took a chemistry class. One day, her professor brought a guest to his lecture. "Ninety percent of you are in this class because it is a pre-med requirement. But there's more to science than medicine. My friend is a chemist who develops new drugs for a pharmaceutical company. He has already helped hundreds of thousands of patients — more than maybe any one doctor ever will." His example opened her eyes to the possibility of a non-medical science career, and she ended up studying biology and child development despite not knowing what she might do with her degree.

Her junior year in college, Priya studied abroad in Italy, where she met her future husband, Fabio, an Italian with a master of fine arts in painting. After traveling around Europe, she returned to the United States for her senior year with wanderlust and a craving for the unfamiliar, intent on finding a meaningful job that would satisfy both.

When she graduated in 1997, Priya took a job supporting family planning and nutrition programs in Africa and Southeast Asia with

John Snow, Inc., a public health management consulting and research firm with offices in Boston and Washington, DC. When she traveled for monthlong monitoring visits to sites to Cambodia she saw a country facing a dire shortage of physicians, rebuilding its health infrastructure after decades of war. "The people were so sick," Priya told me, "and as a public health consultant, even with the best of intentions, there was nothing I could do to help them." Her resolve to find another career besides medicine started to crack. Within a year, she enrolled in night classes to finish her pre-medical requirements, and in the summer of 1999, she wrote her medical school admission essay on a flight to Cambodia.

About the time Priya submitted her application, the grant supporting her work at John Snow ended, and she took a six-month consulting position supporting the Reproductive Health Association of Cambodia. She wanted to continue working with two influential mentors she'd met through John Snow, Ouk Vong Vathiny, MD, the organization's executive director, and Maggie Huff-Rousselle, PhD, the president of Social Sectors Development Strategies, a Massachusetts-based consulting and research company specializing in public health.

Dr. Vathiny told Priya about the plight of doctors in Cambodia after the civil war in the early 1970s. She was in medical school in April 1975 when the Khmer Rouge, led by Pol Pot, invaded Phnom Penh, overthrew the government, and launched a genocidal campaign to reshape the country into a self-sufficient nation of farmers. Soldiers gathered Dr. Vathiny and her classmates in an auditorium, executed their professors in front of them, then sent the students to the countryside to work as farmhands. By the time the country was liberated by the Vietnamese in 1979, just 32 of the 532 physicians practicing in the early 1970s remained. The others had been executed or died doing hard labor in deplorable conditions.[3] Dr. Vathiny then returned to Phnom Penh to finish medical school, becoming a leading voice for reproductive health in the country, which was soon ravaged by the AIDS epidemic of the 1980s.

Dr. Vathiny embodied the notion of "soft power" — a physically beautiful, gentle woman who could be charmingly, almost flirtatiously persuasive one minute, then don her reading glasses and transform into a fierce advocate for marginalized populations, like women in commercial sex work. Change did not happen because of individual or policy-level efforts alone; it always required both. Priya watched Dr. Vathiny teach female sex workers to protect themselves from HIV by deftly applying condoms during oral sex, then later that same day advocate to legislators for broad access to birth control medications and devices.

In Maggie Huff-Rousselle, a consultant to the association, Priya found a model for effective organizational leadership. Huff-Rousselle was a teen mother who founded her own company and earned several advanced degrees. "I learned more from watching her lead and support others than perhaps anyone else ever," Priya recalled, adding that Huff-Rousselle taught her the value of persistence, focusing her actions, finding good partners, and speaking from her heart, not just her head, when working for change.

After a few months with Dr. Vathiny, Priya was sure she wanted to go to medical school but still hadn't told her parents she'd applied, because she didn't want to let them down if she wasn't accepted. During a layover in Indonesia, on her way to Cambodia for what would be her last trip, she found her acceptance letter to Temple University Medical School waiting in her inbox. She immediately called her parents and told them everything. After their initial shock, they were overjoyed. Not only was she following in their footsteps, but she would finally be living close to home again.

In August 2000, Priya moved to Philadelphia to begin medical school. She knew it would take some time to readjust to an academic environment after three years away from school, but her first year was rougher than she expected. Seeing healthcare through Dr. Vathiny's eyes, against the backdrop of a war-torn environment, had sharpened her appreciation for the seriousness and the privilege of her studies, and she struggled to identify with her classmates, mostly recent college graduates with less life experience.

When second year rolled around and things didn't improve, Priya wondered if medicine might not be right for her after all. During the fall, she felt so ambivalent that she took four days off from fall classes, daring herself to quit. For three days, she was happier at home. By the fourth day, she was curious about what she was missing, and on the fifth day she returned to the auditorium, resolved to get through the rest of second year. She hoped the firsthand healing of third-year rotations would be more engaging than memorizing a barrage of dry facts.

Her rotations started in July, and after obstetrics, psychiatry, and surgery, Priya was relieved she'd stuck it out. As third year went on, she found herself most fascinated with the acute phase of disease — she wanted to make the diagnosis and manage the crisis, not watch events play out over years. She liked the way the emergency room boiled medicine to its essence: a patient in need, a doctor to help. The work was also well suited to her interest in public health. As she described in a talk she gave at a regional TEDx conference in 2018, "emergency departments have a unique perspective on the needs of the communities they serve."[4] Priya had found her specialty.

The Temple University Hospital is in a low-income, high-crime neighborhood in North Philadelphia, where many patients are uninsured and often don't come in for care until their diseases are quite advanced. Her attendings didn't sugarcoat any of the realities for the students; nor did they flinch in their care for patients. They also made sure students saw patients whose history or presentation offered a rich learning experience.

Where her attendings weren't as strong was in setting their work in a larger context. When Priya shared observations about the structural causes of their patients' poor health, her perspective was met with: "Public health is for people who can't hack it in real medicine." Not one to accept being easily dismissed, Priya decided to add formal training in public health to her medical degree, to learn how to advocate effectively for policy changes on behalf of her patients.

Between her third and fourth years of medical school, Priya attended Johns Hopkins Bloomberg School of Public Health for a master of public health degree. That fall, she married Fabio, and he finally moved to the United States. After a year of making the two-hour trek between Philadelphia and Baltimore, Priya returned to Temple for her final year of medical school. She stayed at Temple for her emergency medicine residency, spent three years rotating through services in and around Philadelphia, and welcomed her first child during her last year of training.

Her first job as an attending, in 2008, was at the Albert Einstein Medical Center, a large, nonprofit teaching hospital in North Philadelphia. Then in 2012, not long after she had her second child, the chair of emergency medicine at Thomas Jefferson University Hospital reached out and invited her to apply for an open position in his department. Jefferson was a bigger organization with a strong academic reputation, and Priya was eager for ample opportunities to practice, teach, and do research. She interviewed, and when Jefferson offered her the job, she accepted.

Shortly after Priya began working as an emergency room attending, overdose deaths began skyrocketing in Philadelphia. Priya and her fellow emergency physicians faced major barriers to saving lives. One was the lack of access to the lifesaving reversal agent naloxone, often sold under the brand name Narcan, due in part to the stigma of opioid addiction and the perception that a rescue agent allowed her patients to use without consequences. Priya pronounced too many patients dead from an overdose who might have lived if naloxone were in the hands of the people close to them. But even if patients came in alive, her hands were tied by state regulations, which didn't allow doctors to offer medication-assisted treatment and addiction services to patients before they were discharged from the emergency room. Priya was stuck watching, helpless, as patients left her emergency room with nowhere to go other than back to the street drugs that brought them to her in the first place. As she described in her TEDx talk:

> Behind the graphs and the numbers and the statistics are people, husbands and wives, someone's child, my neighbors. I have pulled them blue and lifeless from cars, I have watched their suffering from the chronic disease that is addiction, I have tried to engage them when their fear has prevented them from even being able to look me in the eye and I have watched the anguish of those who love them not know how to help anymore.[5]

Her first goal was to make naloxone more available on the street. In her free time, Priya gave interviews to reporters from the *Philadelphia Inquirer* and other media outlets, testified before the city council, and educated state lawmakers one-on-one.[6] In 2012, she joined a grass-roots coalition, the Philadelphia Emergency Department Prescription Opioid Misuse Working Group, made up of twenty-six representatives from almost every emergency department in the city. After two years of lobbying, the Pennsylvania State General Assembly passed Act 139 on Tuesday, September 30, 2014, allowing anyone to purchase naloxone, even without a physician's prescription, as part of a standing order. Priya described the contributions of the working group in an article for the *Philadelphia Inquirer*.

> Starting as early as 2015, Jefferson and emergency departments across the city started implementing routine naloxone prescribing with discharge from the emergency department to increase access to lifesaving overdose prevention. When we recognized the fleeting moments we have with patients after reversing a near-fatal overdose, some of us worked to develop and advocate for warm hand-off processes to facilitate steps to treatment immediately from the emergency department.

Others developed processes to start medication-assisted treatment with buprenorphine straight away in the hospital, giving a patient some relief and hope while they take the first steps to recovery.

In late 2016, Philadelphia mayor Jim Kenney formed an opioid epidemic task force and offered Priya one of the eighteen seats, based on the work she'd already done and her reputation for elevating the voices of her patients. She joined the commissioners of public health, behavioral health, police, fire, and prison as the only practicing physician in the group. After three months of weekly meetings, Mayor Kenney and Governor Tom Wolf announced the task force report and its long list of recommendations in May 2017. The recommendations formalized the work begun years before by the grassroots coalition that had first changed both opioid and naloxone prescribing patterns.

Satisfied that acting on the changes outlined in the task force report was now in the hands of legislators, Priya saw the lull as a chance to take care of herself. In December 2017, she had pain-relieving surgery she'd put off for almost three years, because her absence from the department, even for a few weeks, would strain her colleagues. At the insistence of her surgeon, she took six weeks off to recover. While at home convalescing, Governor Wolf declared the opioid crisis a statewide public health emergency: "I am using every tool at my disposal to get those suffering from substance use disorders into treatment, save more lives, and improve response coordination."[7] The declaration made naloxone more widely available — first responders could dispense it at the scene of a call, and prisons could give it to at-risk individuals on release — and hospitals and emergency rooms could now start medication-assisted treatment. The Pennsylvania Department of Human Services also launched an incentive program, offering hospitals up to $193,000 to adopt recommendations making it easier to get patients into treatment after an emergency room visit, and for proof that those measures reduced relapse. Priya was proud of the difference she and her colleagues had made for their community and relieved that she could take better care of her patients.

Just about a year after her surgery, Priya left Jefferson, but she declined to discuss why. Since she had otherwise been so forthcoming, I found the omission curious, so I did a little digging and turned up a wrongful termination suit she filed against Jefferson. The text, which is available online, stated that on her first day back from leave, Priya was notified her contract would not be renewed.[8] When I asked Priya about the suit, she acknowledged it was settled out of court in June 2022 but declined to comment further.

Though I can't say for sure, I suspect Priya's experience at Jefferson was like that of most physicians who try to stand up to corporate healthcare, only to realize they have very few rights. Because physicians sign "at will" employment contracts that stipulate they can be fired at any time and for no reason, when they speak up about poor working conditions or impediments to care — unreasonable or unethical performance measures, unsafe staffing levels, workplace discrimination — they can lose their jobs. If they file suit, it may take years to go to trial. During this time they may be unemployed, because of unproven rumors that they are troublemakers, or because of non-compete clauses in their contracts that prevent them from working elsewhere in the region. When the corporation's lawyers offer a settlement, most jump at the chance to put the suit behind them and escape financial limbo, even though accepting a payout usually means agreeing not to disclose the terms of the deal or to disparage the defendants. Unfortunately, such a settlement creates no legal precedent on which the next doctor, similarly wronged, can base a case.[9]

Having only ever worked in academic, urban, high-volume trauma centers, Priya decided to look for a job that would offer her a new challenge. When she visited Jennersville to interview, the bucolic setting soothed her, and though she'd always thought of herself as belonging to urban places, she felt at home in the West Grove community. The hospital didn't have the academic prestige of her previous jobs, or the breadth of services, medical or otherwise, but her team could hold their own, as she wrote in the *Philadelphia Inquirer* in 2020: "The cohort of nurses in the emergency department carried a work ethic and experience base that were unmatched in the hospital as a whole. They knew the responsibilities they bore as a result of their geography and no other backup." Priya relished the challenges her new job at Jennersville offered. "I had to learn a new way of thinking and functioning as a clinician, far from the many services and specialties I had taken for granted. I never thought I would silently pray for no wind and good weather while stabilizing a patient whose aorta was tearing, knowing that a helicopter ride out to a cardiothoracic or vascular surgeon was their only chance of survival."[10]

She was just coming up on her first work anniversary when the coronavirus pandemic hit in March 2020. Nine months later, in December 2020, the layoffs started. Priya was let go in March 2021, and by the summer, the hospital had only a skeleton staff. How was it that even as the third, fourth, and fifth waves of a global pandemic rolled in, healthcare workers at Jennersville — and at so many similar small hospitals around the country — anxiously awaited pink slips?

I learned about the Jennersville Hospital saga from an article Priya published in the *Philadelphia Inquirer* in January 2022. By that point, I'd been working on this book for a year, and I'd read about dozens of hospitals around the country, in small, often rural communities, that had met the same fate. I'd also read scores of articles by physicians frustrated with the decisions of their health systems. But it was rare to find a physician writing about how a closure impacted the community. Priya's piece drew me in because it was fierce and heartfelt, and it resonated with my own perspective. In JENNERSVILLE ISN'T JUST ANOTHER SHUTTERED HOSPITAL. IT WAS MY HOME FOR 2 YEARS, Priya wrote:

> The story of Jennersville Hospital illustrates the complexities
> and far-reaching impacts of valuing "margins over missions"

— or putting profits before patients. As a result of this practice, I have watched highly skilled colleagues walk away from
hospital-based work. I have listened as patients rationalize
their decisions not to seek care earlier due to difficulties and
distance in access. I have felt the forceful ripples of fewer
available inpatient beds all the way back in my Philly emergency department.

Will our leaders, government agencies, medical societies,
and elected officials heed the lessons that Jennersville Hospital offers? Will we understand that the health of the community is not a commodity easily fit into capital markets and
financial models with zero-sum bottom lines, or fodder for
private equity? Until we do, the stories and the voices from
within the hospitals must continue to highlight the issues of
the community and providers who care for them.[11]

After reading her article, I immediately reached out, eager to compare
experiences and think together about how to empower communities to
recognize and speak out about their betrayal by corporate healthcare.

Jennersville is a small subdivision of the village of Penn Township
in Chester County, in southeast Pennsylvania. A graduate of the
University of Pennsylvania, Dr. William B. Ewing, established the
hospital with five beds in 1900. The community was spurred to expand
the facility, reaching into their own pockets to do it, after watching
their neighbors suffer in the pandemic of 1918. Then in 1957, the town
received $180,000 from the Hill Burton Act, federal funding designed
to encourage building and modernization of hospitals, which together
with $900,000 of donations from the community enabled them to
build a new facility that was state-of-the-art for the time.[12] That hospital, only slightly updated, was where Priya worked for two years.

Nonprofit community hospitals like West Grove were never meant
to address every healthcare need. They offered care for common conditions and provided basic lifesaving interventions — establishing an

airway, controlling bleeding, providing circulatory support — to stabilize patients for safe transfer to larger facilities and specialized care. But over the decades, reimbursement shifted to favor specialty care and the basics stopped paying well enough to keep these hospitals alive.

By the late 1990s, West Grove, which by then had changed its name to Southern Chester County Medical Center, suffered an $8 million operating loss after years of rocky finances, and the board of trustees decided it was time to sell to a larger system.[13] Twenty-two potential buyers sent in bids, split equally between for-profit and not-for-profit entities, and in 2001 the board accepted a $20 million offer from Community Health Systems, a for-profit health system.[14] As a nonprofit, West Grove had been exempted from state and local taxes; selling to a for-profit corporation would generate millions in tax revenue for the county's schools, infrastructure, and services.

Community Health Systems also agreed to invest $30 million in improvements to radiology, the laboratory, and the operating rooms and to add another fifty-two beds if the facility met financial targets. Finally, they promised to keep the hospital open for at least a decade, operating under the name Jennersville Regional Hospital.

Fifteen years later, Community Health Systems was $15 billion in debt and floundering.[15] The corporation, which owned 130 hospitals in twenty states,[16] had never recovered from its merger with Health Management Associates in 2014, and its small hospitals were rapidly losing market share to regional consolidation. In 2017, Community Health started a yearslong "portfolio rationalization and deleveraging strategy," colloquially known as a fire sale, to unload the hospitals that were trailing in market share in their respective regions, including five in southeastern Pennsylvania: Jennersville, Brandywine, Phoenixville, Chestnut Hill, and Pottstown Hospitals.

Meanwhile Reading Hospital, an hour from Philadelphia and fifty minutes due north of Jennersville, wanted to expand its network beyond the several physician offices and urgent care centers it owned to increase its leverage in negotiations with insurers. Reading was far enough from the Philadelphia healthcare systems that its customer base had remained strong through years of regional consolidation; in 2016 it had cash reserves of $200 million.[17] With help from global consulting firm McKinsey & Company, Reading executives drafted a plan to build two small hospitals and expand urgent care options in their region. The plan assumed clinicians at the small hospitals would send lucrative outpatient referrals to specialists at Reading and fill the larger hospital's inpatient beds.

Community Health's decision to sell their five hospitals in southeastern Pennsylvania changed Reading's plan. By buying existing hospitals, the system could expand immediately. Reading's CEO consulted advisers, including an investment bank, a law firm, and a consulting group, and made an offer, which Community Health accepted. On Friday, September 29, 2017, Reading closed the $423 million deal. The system was renamed Tower Health and included the five Community Health facilities, the flagship Reading Hospital, a rehabilitation hospital, physician groups, urgent care offices, a surgery center, and a health insurance plan in partnership with University of Pittsburgh Medical Center.[18] Almost immediately, though, Tower Health executives realized two potentially fatal errors. Community Health had deferred tens of millions of dollars in facility repairs and equipment upgrades that required immediate attention, and the five hospitals had to transition to Reading's electronic medical records system, which would cost another $125 million.[19]

The deal also came at a significant cost to the community. When Tower bought Jennersville, the hospital reverted to nonprofit status and was again exempt from paying property taxes. The county relied on the additional funding, especially for its school district, and the budget cuts had an immediate effect. Moreover, Tower Health's strategic plan assumed patients from the smaller hospitals would seek specialty care at Reading. But Reading is nearly twice as far from Jennersville as the internationally renowned Philadelphia hospitals, like Penn and Jefferson, and patients resented feeling even the subtlest pressure to travel farther for care. Their main concern was to be at the hospital closest to their families. When Priya offered her Jennersville patients a referral or transfer to Reading, they often refused, and patients at the other small hospitals in the system did the same.

Over the next two and a half years, the small hospitals lost hundreds of millions of dollars. Then the pandemic hit, and Governor Wolf shut down all but essential care. Demand for services across the Tower Health system dropped 30 to 50 percent overnight, and revenue was down 40 percent. By the end of the second quarter of 2020, the system had lost $212 million; in response, Tower laid off one thousand of its twelve thousand employees.[20] At the end of the third quarter, Tower started trying to sell off its satellite hospitals and urgent care centers, but the big systems knew it was financial suicide to buy distressed community hospitals in the middle of a pandemic, and none of them bid. A year later, in September 2021, Tower reported operating losses of $415 million for the previous fiscal year and announced that if it did not find a buyer by December 2021, Jennersville Hospital would close.[21]

Yet more trouble was brewing for Tower Health. Chester County officials, smarting from lost tax revenue, had paid close attention to Tower Health's business practices and argued they did not accord with its nonprofit status, citing high executive salaries and bonuses based on financial performance. In 2021, the county assessed Tower as a for-profit corporation, levying millions in tax liabilities. Tower appealed the change, which Chester County judge Jeffrey Sommer denied in October 2021, noting scarce evidence that the hospitals were behaving as charitable institutions — the hospitals did not provide sufficient free care, and their business dealings were inextricably linked to, and influenced by, for-profit entities. Moreover, Tower was not operating "free of profit motive," as required of a charitable organization, since executives were paid and incentivized like for-profit executives.[22] Their millions in tax liabilities would stand.

Finally, in November 2021, an offer came from Canyon Atlantic Partners, which calls itself a "hospital turnaround firm,"[23] to buy Jennersville and Brandywine for $16.5 million. They offered just $1 million up front and $11 million to be paid in monthly installments over the subsequent five years. Canyon would pay Tower an additional $4.5 million dollars if the hospital were sufficiently profitable; it would invest at least $5 million in the two hospitals during its first three years of ownership; and would operate the facilities as hospitals for at least two years.[24]

The founder and CEO of Canyon Atlantic, David Kreye, spent fifteen years leading a series of small, for-profit hospitals, including a stint at a Naples, Florida, HMA hospital. When he joined the Naples hospital, he acknowledged his transience while defending his reputation to the local newspaper. "I've taken ailing hospitals and made them successful,"[25] he boasted. The truth is more complicated. He failed to turn around at least two struggling organizations, which forfeited loans or went bankrupt soon after he departed.[26] Nevertheless, Kreye's spotty credentials didn't stop an investment bank from backing his fledgling hospital management corporation when he founded it in 2017.

Chester County leaders cared less about Kreye's weak track record than they did about the immediate fallout of hospital closures. If Jennersville closed, so would Medic 94. With fewer ambulances available and each call requiring a forty-mile round trip to the nearest emergency room — taking them out of the response pool for two hours or more with every call — patients in West Grove might wait two or three times longer for an ambulance to arrive in an emergency. Brandywine was also the primary psychiatric hospital caring for adolescents and patients with eating disorders in the region. As the indigent and elderly from Chester County filled beds at other hospitals, their safe discharge harder to arrange from farther away, the beds they occupied couldn't be used for patients after elective surgery. Without beds, those elective procedures would be delayed, threatening the financial health of other regional hospitals. If Canyon Atlantic bought Jennersville and Brandywine, the whole region could stop holding its breath.

Three weeks after it announced the planned sale, Tower abruptly backed out of the deal, citing concerns about Canyon's financial, regulatory, and operational preparedness to assume ownership.[27] On Friday, December 31, 2021, less than two decades after the board sold it to an outside business interest, Jennersville Hospital closed, probably for good. A hospital grown in one global pandemic died in another.

As anticipated, the closures sent shock waves through the community, as surrounding hospitals strained to absorb the additional volume of patients in the middle of yet another coronavirus surge. A child psychiatrist friend in Philadelphia confessed in February 2022 that she worried every day for her patients who no longer had Brandywine as a nearby option for hospitalization and whose already suffering families would endure additional hardships when they traveled farther to seek care. For six weeks after the closures, Matt Ramsey from chapter 1 canceled dozens of surgeries because his Jefferson satellite hospital, thirty miles from Jennersville, was overwhelmed and out of beds.

When the Jennersville community sold its hospital, it trusted the buyer would maintain the original mission of caring for the community. But Community Health Systems did not answer to the people of Chester County, it answered to distant shareholders. And managing at a distance from the community means those who suffer are no longer neighbors, friends, and business acquaintances; their pain becomes faceless and their needs hypothetical.

Priya watched the final demise of Jennersville from afar. After she was laid off, she went to work for a for-profit emergency physician group that contracts with a for-profit hospital. She has concerns about the model, but she doesn't know what else to do. She's tried just about all the other options in the region. After losing two jobs in the middle of the biggest public health crisis in a century, she no longer trusts the long-recited rhetoric about medicine as a stable career. "I've worked so hard to get here," she confessed in one candid moment, "and now that I'm here, it makes me sick."

Priya spends two mornings a week at her kitchen table with her laptop, after her children leave for school, writing about the ongoing opioid crisis made worse by COVID, about empowering women in the workplace, racial and gender inequity, and public health. Sometimes she is drafting an article for the *Philadelphia Inquirer*, where she is a regular opinion contributor. Other days she works on academic articles for medical journals. She gives problems a human face, illustrating the shortcomings of corporate healthcare by talking about patients like Ms. May, who came into the emergency room with a headache and high blood pressure after two weeks of trying, in vain, to get her doctors' office, pharmacy, and health insurance plan to help renew a prescription. In her TEDx talk, she explained how she arrived at this strategy.

> When it became clear that the stories of Ms. May were not being heard at higher levels, I became acutely aware of my greater responsibility. This has driven me to expand my efforts outside the walls of the emergency department. How could I use [what] I've learned in the emergency department to increase health equity? How could I show others the phenomenal potential of capitalizing on the reach and access of the emergency department to help impact the health of a community? How could I make the emergency department a tool of social justice?

Priya knows change is hard, but living without trying means succumbing to her moral injury, becoming callous and broken and betraying her colleagues and patients in turn. As she said herself, in that same 2018 talk, "power belongs to the problem solvers."

I interpret the world through the lens of an emergency
physician but also as a public health advocate, as a member
of the Philadelphia community, as the daughter of immigrants, as a wife and a mother, as a supporter of the fundamental rights to equal access to care. I am a believer in the
power of urban resilience and social justice to increase and
improve the future for all of us . . . the cavalry may not be
coming and even if they do, they will not see what we see
from the frontlines of our world. It starts with us. We have
the power to disrupt for greater good. We can change our
world. Power belongs to the problem solvers.

CHAPTER NINE

Costs and Benefits

On Friday, January 13, 2017, my husband's congenital heart condition, which had been stable for years, abruptly deteriorated. Drowning in fluid building up in his lungs, Shervin was admitted to a local hospital, where he stayed for several days while doctors waited for the situation to resolve. Though his condition continued to deteriorate, the doctors balked at changing treatment plans and prickled when I raised the question of a transfer. By the time they admitted they couldn't manage his care, his situation was dire.

We planned to transfer Shervin by air ambulance to the Mayo Clinic in Rochester, Minnesota, where specialists well versed in his rare condition had been treating him for years. While waiting at his bedside for word about when the ambulance would arrive, a woman from the billing office appeared. Consulting her clipboard, she explained that before the hospital would transfer him, I had to accept full responsibility for paying his costs out-of-pocket if our "best possible" insurance refused to pay. A quirk of how Mayo Clinic billed, combined with caveats in our coverage, left us at risk.

The woman couldn't tell me who, exactly, required my guarantee, how much we were talking about, or who could provide further clarification. All I knew was that if I didn't agree, Shervin couldn't be transferred, and if he wasn't transferred, he probably wouldn't survive. And every minute I took to understand the implications of what I was signing delayed his transfer. To save my husband, I would have to sign a blank check and hope it didn't ruin us.

I asked her for a minute to collect some information.

While my husband struggled for every breath, I stepped into an alcove in the hallway so I could spare him the brutality of my next conversation. A quick calculation, based on work I'd recently done on surgery costs after transplants — a heart transplant was the very worst-case scenario, but one he was inching closer to every hour — estimated our potential bill at nearly $1 million including an air ambulance, operating room costs, and weeks in intensive care. I called our financial planner and asked whether a hospital bill that size would be financially ruinous for us. While I waited for him to review our accounts, my mind spun through the consequences of paying a bill like that. Would we lose our home? Our eldest had just started college — would he be able to finish where he started? Would our youngest even have a college fund, or would we need to raid that to keep his father alive? And if Shervin survived, how much would he resent me for keeping him alive but losing everything we had worked decades to build and for robbing our children of their opportunities?

Finally, our financial planner came back on the line and gave me a number. Swallowing hard, I returned to Shervin's bedside and signed the paper. It would be a close scrape, but we could swing it. We had just paid off our medical school loans; if we needed to borrow again, we would. This time, I could save him without ruining us. But what would happen next time, or to my friends and neighbors who weren't doctors, well versed in the costs and complexities of the business of healthcare, if they were ever on the spot to make a call like this?

Too often what happens is that people lose everything. A Kaiser Family Foundation / *New York Times* survey in 2016 found that insurance provides only modest protection; 20 percent of people with insurance, whether public or private, carried medical debt, compared with 53 percent of those who are uninsured. Worse yet, two-thirds of those bills were due to a single event, not from managing a chronic illness.[1] In 2017, 19 percent of US households received medical bills they could not immediately pay off in full.[2] A 2019 study on medical bankruptcy by David Himmelstein, a professor in the School of

Public Health at City University of New York, found that two-thirds of personal bankruptcies are in some way tied to medical debt, either because of the bills themselves, or due to lost wages of the person in the household who needed care, or the one who had to stop working to become a caregiver.[3] "The insurance that is available and affordable to people, or that most people's employers provide them," the study concluded, "is not adequate protection if you're sick."[4]

The next morning as Shervin was readied for transfer, the storm I'd been watching for two days hit, grounding flights across the Midwest. For hours, the jet ambulance sat on the tarmac in Minnesota, waiting for clearance to fly to Pennsylvania and back; at two in the afternoon, the dispatcher called my mobile to tell me they were giving up, his voice unsteady as he delivered the news that might seal my husband's fate. After scrambling for a new plan and asking favors of a hand transplant colleague connected with the heart transplant team at the University of Pennsylvania, a ground ambulance took Shervin on a midnight run to Penn, two hours away in Philadelphia. One of the cardiologists who cared for him there had trained with Shervin's team at Mayo, and within twenty-four hours of starting a new treatment plan, his condition improved dramatically. He came home ten days later, feeling well for the first time in six months.

To my enormous relief, our insurance never questioned Shervin's bills, but our close brush with financial insolvency, despite carrying the best insurance offered, left me deeply unsettled. The rhetoric often recited by hospital business offices is that patients must be more responsible for their own finances if they wished to avoid insolvency. But what if their insurance is intentionally indecipherable, or if they are too ill to grapple with its complexity?

The term *financial toxicity* was coined in the early 2010s "to bring attention to the high costs of cancer treatments and the resulting financial burden and distress on patients and their families."[5] Since then, as treatment innovations, with associated high costs, have crept into other areas of medicine, increasing numbers of patients with cardiovascular, lung, or joint diseases are facing crippling bills. As Susan Gubar, a patient with ovarian cancer, wrote in the *New York Times*, "cancer treatment escalates the possibility of penury, and treatment-produced fiscal catastrophes are tied to cancer deaths. . . . What aims to save us can destroy us."[6]

Online platforms have become virtual doctors' lounges as the real ones have disappeared. They are places where doctors can get all manner of guidance from colleagues in diverse specialties around the country, from real-time updates about symptoms and treatments in the earliest days of COVID to suggestions for managing employment and reimbursement challenges. In June 2021, shortly after I started writing this book, I was on one such forum, skimming through comments about who bore responsibility for the costs of care, when Dr. Blake Alkire's comment in defense of patients caught my eye.

Blake, an ear, nose, and throat surgeon at Massachusetts Eye and Ear Infirmary, a hospital affiliated with Harvard University, wrote, "Very few people understand the true mechanics of how their insurance works — including many doctors." To support his point, he referenced a study by the Kaiser Family Foundation of people with employer-sponsored health insurance; 44 percent of participants said they have a hard time knowing how much of their treatment costs they are responsible for, and 40 percent of people said it is difficult to understand what's covered by their insurance.[7]

Moreover, Dr. Alkire wrote, recent research by his colleagues found that not all patients are willing to go bankrupt to cure what ails them.[8] But patients can only make informed decisions if their doctors take the time to explain the consequences of each potential course of action, including the financial effects. I responded privately, asking whether he thought inflicting financial toxicity might be a form of moral injury. His response was immediate, and the emphasis is his:

> I cite the article — now movement — that you and Simon authored **all** the time. I had never thought about this as a

source of moral injury, but now it is abundantly clear to me that it is. Try as I might to prevent billing surprises, it still happens to my patients way too often. Because I feel a moral obligation to ensure that patients are not financially devastated for the care I provide (especially because almost everything I deal with is elective), I ask patients to let me know about any surprise or unexpected bills. When they do, I can usually waive my charges, but the hospital of course does not budge [on its fees]. There are a few folks who I have lost sleep over given their precarious financial well-being . . . I want to rescue my patients and know that, ethically, I can't personally pay for their care, but the intuition to do so speaks to the psychic pain of bearing responsibility for expressly violating our oath to do no harm.

That online exchange was the first of many conversations I had with Blake about his efforts to address financial toxicity. Growing up the son of an orthopedic surgeon in a small, tight-knit community, Blake never imagined he might face such a dilemma when he became a doctor — unwittingly harming patients, financially, while he healed them physically.

Blake grew up in Texarkana, a city of about thirty-six thousand at the far northeastern edge of Texas, where Oklahoma, Louisiana, and Arkansas converge. His grandfather, a pilot who was captured and held as a prisoner of war during World War II, believed his faith saved him, and he gave generously to his church, both in time and in treasure; as a result, family members were, as Blake put it, "second pew Methodists."

His father, Chris, traveled to remote areas in South America every year to provide charity orthopedic care, performing simple surgeries — a carpal tunnel release, a ganglion cyst removal, or a club foot repair — that dramatically improved the patient's quality of life. When Blake was a teenager, he joined his father on these trips; though current ethics in global health would preclude such participation today, at the time it was normal for doctors to bring their children along.

In one of our first conversations, Blake shared a vivid memory of his father counseling a young surgeon who was on his first international medical trip about treatment decisions in global health. The young surgeon wanted to do a complex tendon transfer, a procedure often done in the United States to help patients with a nerve injury that causes foot drop. Chris patiently reminded his young colleague what that surgery entailed: four hours in the operating room, and four people on staff — two surgeons, a nurse, and an anesthetist. After surgery the patient couldn't bear weight on that leg for twelve weeks, which for someone who does manual labor would mean not working. Moreover, the surgery would fail if the patient did not follow up with months of physical therapy, and there were no physical therapists in this remote location.

In the same four hours in the operating room, the two surgeons could instead cure at least sixteen patients of carpal tunnel syndrome, Dupuytren's contractures, or ganglion cysts. On these trips, Chris explained, they aimed to do the greatest good for the greatest number, which meant they sometimes had to make the painful, but necessary, decision not to do some surgeries. Just because something could be done didn't always mean it was the right thing to do.

Blake remembers looking out at the Andes from the hospital where he spent his third trip, and knowing, without making a conscious decision, that he would become a doctor and spend at least part of his time working in other countries. He wanted to relieve suffering and medicine seemed like the most immediate, direct, and personal way to do it. In that moment, he committed to his career path.

After earning his undergraduate degree in cellular and molecular biology, with a minor in piano, at Vanderbilt, Blake went to Harvard Medical School. In recent years funders had begun pressuring global health groups to move beyond heartwarming humanitarian stories and prove the economic value of their work. Between his third and fourth years of medical school, Blake decided to study for a master of public health degree, also at Harvard, which set his work in the context of global social and economic issues and prepared him to conduct the kind of research funders demanded.

Although Blake was drawn to the fast, sure fixes of surgical interventions, he worried his contemplative and forgiving temperament was a poor fit for such a hard-charging field. During a brief rotation in his third year on the ENT (ear, nose, and throat) service, Blake was struck by the compassion shown by ENT residents and attendings to their patients and students alike. A monthlong fourth-year elective confirmed that the specialty was a good match. The attendings patiently explained, sometimes repeatedly, diagnoses and plans to their patients. They coached Blake on pathophysiology and anatomy and taught him the physics behind radiology studies — not just how to interpret the images but also how they were created — so he could pick up aberrations in technique. ENT surgery was also well suited to global health work because they did short, simple procedures that provided immediate symptom relief or improved function, like cochlear implants to improve hearing and sinus surgery to reduce painful infections. Blake had found his career.

But before graduating and starting his residency, Blake spent a year doing research with Dr. John Meara, who founded Harvard's Program in Global Surgery and Social Change, exploring how society benefits when individuals in the developing world undergo plastic and neurosurgery interventions.[9] Correcting disfigurement, for example, allowed people to enter the workforce more easily, making their society more productive. As part of his research, he tried to identify the age at which the best outcome intersected with the lowest cost of repairing a cleft lip, a common disfigurement.[10] During that year, Blake also applied for residency spots.

Hoping to train with the same team that was so committed and kind, Blake ranked the Harvard ENT surgery program first on his match list; staying at Harvard would also mean he could continue his research from his master's degree without having to start over with a different team. Harvard, likewise, ranked Blake at the top of their match list. During his next four years in Boston, Blake juggled the dual demands of training and high-intensity research, with little time for much else.

During Blake's residency, the World Health Organization announced a goal of eliminating medical impoverishment by 2030. In response, *The Lancet*, an esteemed British journal of medicine, launched a Commission on Global Surgery to study how surgical and anesthesia care could improve "the health of individuals and the economic productivity of countries" and invited global health luminaries like Drs. Atul Gawande and Paul Farmer to participate. His mentor Dr. Meara, a classmate and friend of Farmer, called Blake and asked if he would like to join the project. Miraculously, the dates of the Lancet commission aligned exactly with Blake's assigned research time in residency, and he eagerly signed on.

The following year, the commission published its landmark initial report, "Global Surgery 2030," presenting "findings on the state of surgical care in low-income and middle-income countries (LMICs), as well as a framework of recommendations, indicators and targets needed to achieve the Commission's vision of universal access to safe, affordable surgical and anesthesia care when needed."[11] Among the findings, one in particular stuck with Blake: Thirty-three million individuals face catastrophic health expenditure due to payment for surgery and anesthesia each year.

During his residency at Massachusetts Eye and Ear, Blake's attendings coached him on his operating skills, his diagnostic acumen, and how to explain complex matters to his patients and their families in language they could understand. They also modeled how to work well with other surgeons, clinically and administratively, by being responsive, respectful, and gracious. And they taught him how to protect himself from litigation. But they rarely talked about what it cost to do their work. In South America, and during trips to West Africa and the Caribbean in medical school and residency, Blake listened to countless debates between surgeons and economists about whether surgery — or recovery — was economically justified or feasible. After his extensive research on the costs and value of surgery around the globe, Blake found the absence of such discussions in the United States puzzling, especially as economic pressures on patients rose.

When Blake tried to find out what the hospital would bill a patient for his services or the tests he ordered, and how much of that bill the insurer would reimburse, he ran into dead ends. Although the Centers for Medicare and Medicaid Services hold physicians responsible for the accuracy of bills sent in their name, hospitals typically require employed physicians to sign over their billing rights. Hospitals claim that physicians are allowed to review bills for accuracy, as is required by law, but in practice, doctors report challenges accessing those bills, and doing reviews is yet one more task to do after hours. Even if Blake did find out what one patient paid for a test or procedure, that price might not apply to someone else. Like at most hospitals, costs at Mass Eye and Ear are considered proprietary information; the health system negotiates separately with each insurer, and rates can vary dramatically.[12]

Patients are uncomfortable discussing costs with their doctors for similar reasons: They don't want to risk subpar care by cutting costs; they think physicians are not the right experts to consult on financial matters; and they may be embarrassed to discuss their financial situation.[13] The question of cost is almost always lurking for patients, though. At hospitals operating under a fee-for-service model — like Massachusetts Eye and Ear — every test generates revenue, so administrators have no incentive to reduce testing. But for patients, copayments can quickly add up to hundreds or thousands of dollars. Every test, whether a biopsy, lumbar puncture, or even a routine colonoscopy, carries risk, especially for those who are fragile, but even for healthy patients. A 2004 study by the Dartmouth Institute for Health

Policy and Clinical Practice found that for most patients, simply getting more services didn't result in better outcomes because the complications inherent in overtesting negated the potential benefits of having more information.[14]

When Blake asked colleagues, informally, about how concerned they were about the costs of testing, he got a variety of responses, all of them truthful and none of them satisfying. Most defended the testing as legitimate, based on sound reasoning and a valid differential diagnosis. Despite the hype about the electronic medical record, previous test results are not always accessible, so patients sometimes need to repeat tests done elsewhere. Like their patients, doctors are also worried about missed diagnoses, but not just because of the patient suffering it would create. An elder statesman of the surgery department often asked his residents, "What's the cost of a missed cancer?" For each one hundred doctors in practice, attorneys file sixty-eight medical liability claims, and more than half of physicians older than fifty-four have been sued. Some specialties, such as general surgery, obstetrics, urology, and ENT, are at particularly high risk, and some states are worse than others — more than 70 percent of physicians in Kentucky, Nevada, and Illinois have been sued, for example.[15] Only 1 percent of the suits that make it to trial are found in favor of the patient-plaintiff, but no one ever knows which one that will be, and defending against a suit is time-intensive and psychologically grueling.[16]

This line of reasoning left Blake feeling trapped. In protecting himself legally, he might unwittingly inflict financial toxicity. But what else could he do?

Surely some patients would opt for a small risk of an inaccurate diagnosis if it left them in a better state of financial health — at the very least, they would want to have an open conversation about their options, like the surgeons did on charity trips in South America. But this hunch was based only on anecdotal observations; Blake had no hard data on the issue in the United States. Moreover, he wasn't yet aware of any colleagues who were similarly conflicted, so when he moved from resident to attending physician at Massachusetts Eye and Ear, where he was hired as clinical faculty, he kept his concerns to himself. Then, just a few months into his practice he saw a young woman who validated his worries and convinced him to look more closely at the problem close to home.

Two years into Blake's practice, he met a patient named Erin. She had already undergone an extensive workup and an expensive procedure at a Fallon Health office in central Massachusetts, but her persistent cough still had not improved, so she came to Massachusetts Eye and Ear for a second opinion. When Blake finished his assessment and made his recommendations, Erin sat quietly for a minute, wringing her hands. "How much will surgery cost here? Because I don't know if I can afford another one." Her previous procedure, she told him, had left her many thousands of dollars in debt, and she was struggling to make the monthly payments while earning just minimum wage. Though Erin had heard of charity care, she had assumed she wouldn't qualify, because she wasn't indigent. She'd heard stories of patients who couldn't pay their bills being sued by hospitals, having their wages garnished, or going bankrupt, and they frightened her. If getting better meant financial ruin, she wasn't sure it would be worth it.

Blake paused for a moment, uncertain how to respond. He didn't know the answer to her question; for that matter, he wasn't even sure where to begin looking for it, other than somewhere in the billing office. He decided to suggest that they delay any next steps — her condition wasn't an emergency — until he could find someone to help them sort out the financial issues. He wanted to be sure his care, and all its consequences, would help Erin more than it hurt her.

After their conversation, Blake didn't know whether to scream or to cry. It seemed almost cruel to dangle treatment in front of patients then leave them alone to decide whether it was truly worthwhile and within their reach, financially. Paradoxically, his patients in sub-Saharan Africa had seemed less distressed when debating whether they could afford a lifesaving procedure than this patient, who theoretically had more resources, here in Boston.

In the days that followed, Blake called the hospital billing office, who pointed him to their financial counselors, who in turn referred him to a financial advocate at a local nonprofit, an expert in negotiating with insurers to reduce medical debt. He connected them with Erin, and they convinced the debt holders to reduce her bills by 85 percent. It was still more than she could comfortably manage at once, but she wouldn't be paying it off for the rest of her life.

For Blake, this encounter with Erin marked a turning point. He was no longer merely flirting with a vague sense of unease; with a thirty-year career stretching out in front of him, he was now terrified that for some of his patients, providing care might inflict harm in the form of financial toxicity, and he wouldn't even know it. To ensure his care was truly helping his patients, Blake would need to learn how to treat them as whole people with multiple, sometimes competing, priorities, including how they preferred to spend their hard-earned money.

The United States spends $11,945 annually per person on healthcare, more than any other country by a wide margin; Switzerland is the next biggest spender at $7,138, and the average for comparable countries is $5,736.[17] Yet patient outcomes in the United States lag behind those of other wealthy countries. Preventable mortality and maternal mortality in the United States, for example, are twice that of comparable countries.[18]

Despite this discrepancy between costs and outcomes, as a society we are squeamish about setting limits on healthcare spending. For decades, researchers have explored ways to control costs, which, despite various attempts to rein them in, continued to rise. By the early 2000s, healthcare made up one-sixth of the United States economy. As President Barack Obama declared at the White House healthcare forum in March 2009, "The biggest threat to our nation's balance sheet is the skyrocketing cost of health care."[19]

In a June 2009 article for *The New Yorker* titled "The Cost Conundrum," Dr. Atul Gawande explored why healthcare costs in McAllen, Texas, were twice the national average.[20] In the article, he compared McAllen to El Paso, a city with similar demographics that spends only half as much on healthcare. The main reason for such high costs in McAllen, he found, was doctors providing "too much" care — ordering too many tests, diagnosing too many marginal conditions, and recommending unnecessarily expensive treatments. Gawande noted that this approach to care was harmful to the people of McAllen, both because of the financial burden of out-of-pocket costs and because of the risks inherent in even the most benign-seeming testing.

In 2010, the Institute of Medicine, which has since been renamed the National Academy of Medicine, published a report declaring that 30 percent of healthcare spending in the United States, about $750 billion, was wasteful. More than half of that waste, the report estimated, was due to unnecessary health services and excess administrative costs.[21] In 2013, the institute issued a follow-up report titled *Best Care at Lower Cost: The Path to Continuously Learning Health Care in America*, shifting the conversation about how to reduce healthcare costs from controlling the volume of care provided to increasing the value of care delivered.[22] The report defined *value* as "the level of benefit achieved for a given cost" and divided care into high-value and low-value categories, intended to guide clinicians to abandon the latter practices.

Each of these publications, among many others, explored the costs to society when one-sixth of the economy was eaten up by healthcare, and how we might legislate and regulate our way to lower costs. But no one had asked the residents of McAllen or El Paso what their own healthcare spending meant to them.

How many people would bankrupt themselves to cure what ailed them? How many would accept some level of risk to avoid financial ruin? The prevailing wisdom in medicine was that individuals facing a potentially lethal disease would opt for a cure at any cost, but this assumption had never been tested. Healthcare systems in the United States demand data for every decision they make, even one as commonsensical as encouraging doctors to talk with patients about their values and their finances before choosing a care option with high out-of-pocket costs. Blake would feel more comfortable changing how he practiced if he had good data to back him up. He turned to his colleague Dr. Mark Shrime, with whom he'd done work on international cost questions, to set up a study of patient preferences in the United States.

Shrime and his colleagues asked 2,359 research subjects to assign a value to treatments for a hypothetically lethal disease that was variably likely to lead to cure and bankruptcy.[23] Just 33 percent of patients chose "cure at all costs." Almost 60 percent of participants had concerns, to varying degrees, about the cost of treatment, and one in twelve people, or 8 percent of participants, said they would choose solvency at all cost — they would rather die of their illness than live having gone bankrupt or otherwise ruined their families financially.

Blake was shocked when he read the results of the study. If this is how people responded in the face of a fatal illness, he reasoned that the numbers would shift even further toward a preference for solvency in patients, like most of his, who had conditions that were nettlesome but not life threatening. When Blake went to his chairman to confess his discomfort, he was relieved to learn the chairman was already discussing his own patients' values and priorities; he just hadn't thought to talk about what he was doing with his colleagues.

Armed with this information, and bolstered by his chair's support, Blake vowed to include patient values in treatment planning. Clinicians looked to places like Harvard for guidance; if doctors there started talking about the issue, changing their own practices, and training residents accordingly, other institutions might follow.

In developing his approach to patient conversations, Blake drew on his experience listening to his father and other clinicians in Ecuador debating how to balance patient goals, constraints, and priorities against likely treatment outcomes. Today, his conversations with patients look a lot like those Matt Ramsey from chapter 1 has with his patients. When he meets them, Blake takes the time to learn who they are as people. What are their interests and hobbies, their sources of joy? Who depends on them every day, and for what? What were their previous experiences like in healthcare? What are their goals for his care? What do they worry about, especially with regard to his care? Do they have concerns about paying for what he might recommend?

After reviewing his diagnosis and treatment plan in detail, Blake explains how to make sense of the finances, providing his patients with billing codes and a primer on how to ask their insurer for a very specific estimate of their costs. If he anticipates that pharmacy costs might be high, he suggests a variety of workarounds: asking what the medication cost would be without using their insurance, comparing prices at other pharmacies, or using a discount prescription service. If patients may meet income criteria, he encourages them to talk with the financial office about discounted or free care at Mass Eye and Ear. Finally, he plainly states he is always open to revising a treatment plan if costs are uncomfortably high. Blake also asks his patients to bring in any bills that surprise them. If he can't make sense of the charges, the patient's responsibility, or how billing works and money flows, he talks to the hospital's financial counselors himself.

As a result of these discussions, his patients sometimes decline certain tests or elect not to have surgery, so his compensation, which is partially "performance-based," is a little lower, and the hospital makes a bit less money. But for Blake, knowing he is truly putting his patients first is worth more than a few thousand dollars in his pocket; thus far, no one has commented that his revenue isn't meeting targets, but if his hospital ever pushed back, he feels protected. Shrime's data supports his position that financial considerations matter to patients, his chairman shares his approach, and his association with global superstars like Paul Farmer and Atul Gawande lends his perspective credibility.

At every opportunity, Blake encourages his colleagues and residents to think beyond performance metrics and treat the whole patient, sharing data and techniques to support them in engaging in conversations about values and finances. He wants to prevent as many doctors as possible from being blindsided by the realization they might be harming patients in their efforts to heal.

Over the past two decades, employers have shifted more costs to patients to encourage "wiser spending," which has brought the issue of price transparency into focus. Patients trying to comparison-shop regularly ran into dead ends trying to get estimates of care costs from hospitals. While I was writing this book, the Hospital Price Transparency rule went into effect. Beginning January 1, 2021, Congress required hospitals to publish prices for the three hundred most common procedures, mostly ones that can be scheduled in advance, both to allow for research and data collection, and to provide patients with information to make cost comparisons when "shopping" for healthcare.

When I asked Blake what he thought about this legislation, he told me he thinks it's an important step in the right direction, but for many patients he's not sure much will change. To get an estimate, patients must know the diagnostic code for their condition and procedure codes for their treatment, as well as the location and the date their procedure will occur. But for most patients, navigating "ICD-10 and CPT" codes is like learning a foreign language, something that is hard enough to do when they are well and close to impossible if they are acutely ill.

Faced with the moral injury of inflicting financial harm on his patients, Blake Alkire acted by changing his practice. Today his practice aligns with his oath to put his patients first, and his leadership supports him. He is keenly aware of the pressures his mentors at other hospitals are under to compromise their practices for the good of their organizations. Blake hopes their examples, and the lessons they've shared with him, will allow him to craft a different future for himself and for those who follow.

CHAPTER TEN

Empowering Physicians

The second I hit the ground on a balmy day in early January 2007, dragged off a trailer by a young horse, I knew I'd dislocated my "good" shoulder. Doctors at the Carlisle Regional Medical Center popped it back in, wished me luck, and suggested I follow up with the local orthopedist, who turned out to be nearing retirement and was more interested in denigrating my hobby than fixing my shoulder. Fortunately, I was already on Dr. Jerry Williams's schedule at the University of Pennsylvania for a second opinion about my "bad" shoulder, so I called to let his office know we might need to talk about both. It took the receptionist a minute to locate my name, as it was on another doctor's list.

Confused, I explained I'd waited two months specifically to see Dr. Williams.

"Dr. Williams is no longer with Penn, though," she said flatly, as if I should have known.

I asked her several questions — when he left, where he went, why I wasn't notified, and whether the other physician was a member of the society of American Shoulder and Elbow Surgeons — none of which she could answer. Sensing my mounting bewilderment and frustration, and no doubt approaching the two-minute time limit most schedulers have with each caller, she offered to change my appointment to see Dr. Matt Ramsey, from chapter 1, the acting chief of the shoulder service. I agreed to the switch, then decided to do some digging. Such an abrupt departure was so unusual that I checked obituaries in Philadelphia and scoured medical publications for news, fear-ing something catastrophic had happened. When I found nothing, I called my mentor from medical school, a shoulder surgeon who had referred me to Dr. Williams, but he, too, was in the dark. Something about the situation didn't add up, but I couldn't figure out just what.

Two weeks later, I met Matt. Though his no-nonsense appraisal of my shoulders took me aback, he clearly had compassion for my situation, so I scheduled surgery for late March, when my husband could be off work to help with childcare. Then, ten days before my surgery, I got a call from a close friend working in orthopedics in North Carolina. "There's a rumor down here that your surgeon's leaving Penn," my friend told me.

Nearing panic — my shoulder was a mess, and I couldn't imagine trying to find another surgeon on short notice — I called Matt's office the next day and left a message. He returned the call himself.

"Word on the street in North Carolina is that you're leaving Penn."

"How reliable was the source?"

"Another shoulder surgeon." Matt was silent. I knew he probably couldn't tell patients he was leaving; most big hospital contracts include a non-solicitation clause that prevents doctors from encouraging patients to follow them to their new practice. When it was clear he wasn't going to say more, I added, "Look, I just need to know if you're moving across town or across the country and how long after my surgery that's going to be."

He assured me he'd be at Penn through my follow-up and that there would be family strife if he suggested moving away. It was his way of telling me, without telling me, that he wasn't leaving the area. It was only in retrospect, during our long conversations for this book, that I realized the sense I had of something being "off" all those years ago was Penn's shoulder service imploding.

A few months before my original appointment, Jerry Williams, Matt, and another surgeon had decided they could not create the kind of shoulder service they envisioned if they stayed at Penn. Among them they had nearly forty years of experience and were experts in maximizing efficiency while maintaining high-quality care: how many patients they could see each day at each level of complexity, how many exam rooms and how many assistants they needed to keep their workflow smooth and orderly. But administrators weren't willing to adapt the standardized system to the particulars of care for shoulder patients. It was time to go somewhere that valued patients enough to appreciate the surgeons' input.

Because he had seniority, Jerry approached the administration first. He wanted to unwind his relationship with Penn carefully and professionally, so he didn't abandon either his patients or his fellows. But starting that conversation unleashed a firestorm.

Every year since he'd started at Penn, Jerry submitted a disclosure of the royalties he received for doing work on his own time, outside of clinical or research obligations to the health system. For fifteen years, the university had acknowledged receipt, but otherwise ignored the disclosures, and never raised the issue in contract renewals; Jerry figured they were tracking numbers to tout in advertising or recruiting efforts.

But now that he was contemplating a move, Penn claimed Jerry owed a substantial portion of those royalties, dating back to his start date. University executives all the way up to the CEO eventually became involved in the dispute. Jerry didn't understand why the issue was only coming up now, but he was willing to compromise both on past royalties and future earnings so they could part on good terms. Penn, for whatever reason, wasn't willing to meet him halfway.

Jerry had dual appointments at the university, which had purview over his academic and research activities, and at the hospital, for his clinical work. His final proposal to leadership, in which he agreed not to pursue legal action against the institution, was to resign from the university immediately, while staying on at the hospital for a few more months until his patients and fellows could smoothly transition to another doctor. Penn accepted his financial terms but terminated both of his appointments, effective the following week.

Jerry was a world-renowned shoulder surgeon, and Penn had just treated him as if he were disposable, putting its own agenda squarely ahead of the needs of his patients and trainees, neither of whom were sufficiently empowered to advocate for themselves. Watching Jerry's saga unfold, Matt and the other surgeon got spooked. They didn't have his clout, his reputation, or his financial cushion. They needed time to reevaluate their own plans and, more immediately, to pick up the pieces from Jerry's hasty exit.

Ten years before the standoff over Jerry's contract, Matt finished his fellowship at Penn and jumped at the chance to stay on as an attending surgeon so he could continue working with Jerry and with Dr. Joseph Iannotti, both legends in the field of shoulder surgery. In addition to being two of the best shoulder surgeons in the country, Drs. Williams and Iannotti were models of personal conduct and servant leadership, who cared equally about their patients, trainees, colleagues, and the future of their field. They were also unrivaled mentors who coached, supported, and championed their trainees to achieve the regional and national recognition they needed to advance their careers. Matt felt they were building the Penn shoulder service into a model of excellent patient care, and he wanted to be part of it.

Matt spent his first five years at Penn finding his footing as an attending surgeon, collecting observations about potential improvements to patient care, watching how his senior partners engaged with administrators about making changes, and identifying the stakeholders and power players he would need to influence if he were to do the same. When he started sharing his ideas with his administration, he recommended approaches that he'd researched thoroughly and thought Penn could implement within the constraints of their systems. With a reputation for speaking up only when he knew what he was talking about and the credibility that came with being an expert surgeon, Matt expected he would find a receptive audience.

He was sorely mistaken. "It felt impossible to ask for changes as a surgeon," he told me. "If it wasn't the administration's idea, it wasn't happening." One of the first things he tried to tackle was scheduling in his clinic, since he was so overbooked that he ran late for almost every appointment after the first few in the morning. Matt went to his administrators and proposed capping the number of patients scheduled each hour, so schedulers couldn't triple-book every appointment time in his clinic, which he thought was an easy fix to improve both patient and physician experience.

Scheduling, it turns out, had its own reasons for maintaining the status quo. Penn was an early adopter of patient satisfaction surveys, which were sent out after appointments or surgery. Each section of the survey singled out a different part of the organization for evaluation, from scheduling to reception to clinicians to parking. High scores won accolades and sometimes bonuses; low scores earned criticism and sometimes even put jobs at risk. Motivated by surveys, scheduling staff wanted patients to remember making their appointment as a pleasant and efficient experience. To that end, schedulers often gave them what they wanted, even if it meant overbooking the surgeons. The packed clinic might run hours behind, but unsuspecting patients would give the schedulers high marks on the survey while rating the surgeon or the clinic staff as slow and disorganized. For their part, department administrators were disinclined to support caps that might impact productivity by reducing the total number of patients Matt could see. He seemed to be managing the workload and though patients grumbled, they kept coming, so their experience couldn't be that bad. Despite repeated efforts, Matt never succeeded in making changes to scheduling at Penn.

The next issue he identified was getting his patients timelier results from imaging. When someone needed an MRI, for instance, they often had to wait a week or two for an appointment, and yet longer for results. Matt needed this information to decide a course of treatment; without it, patients were stuck in limbo. He tried to get radiology to hold a few slots open for same-day orthopedics appointments, because he knew he could fill them every day, but administrators dismissed that idea, too. Radiology had its own productivity targets to meet, and they preferred the certainty of fully booking the schedule in advance.

Most frustrating was his inability to convince the administration to establish dedicated teams for surgery. Each time Matt operated at Penn, he worked with a different surgical team, drawn from the dozens of nurses, technicians, and anesthesiologists on staff. Though each individual was highly skilled, if they didn't rotate through orthopedics regularly, and through the shoulder service in particular, their knowledge wasn't current. Whenever he operated, he lost precious time explaining patient positioning, anticipating next steps, or waiting for instruments or materials because staff couldn't stay one step ahead. Every time the flow paused, even for a second, it added time to the operation, and it took effort to get back in sync. It also increased his cognitive burden, so his days were more physically and mentally draining than they had to be.

Matt had read about emerging evidence from a variety of fields — medicine, aviation, information technology, sports — showing that teams with even modest experience working together enjoy significant advantages.[1] One study of software teams found that groups who worked together 50 percent more often made 20 percent fewer mistakes and went off budget 30 percent less often.[2]

According to his research, the dedicated team would ideally consist of everyone involved in a patient's surgery, from the front door to the recovery room. But even just keeping the same people in the operating room with the surgeon each time they operate — the scrub nurse, operating room technician, circulating nurse, and ideally the anesthesiologist — dramatically improves team performance. When team members are familiar with one another, and with the types of cases the surgeon routinely performs, the surgery goes faster. Quicker surgery is better for patients as it means less time under anesthesia and a lower risk of postoperative nausea and vomiting, blood clots, infections, and other complications. A study of spinal surgery in children found that dedicated teams reduced operative time by nearly one-third, from 395 minutes to 317;[3] another study found the time patients spent in the operating room was on average 13 minutes shorter, reduced from 125 minutes to 112.

Working more efficiently wasn't just good for patients, Matt argued each time he made his case to administrators, it was also good for the bottom line. In 2014 it cost, on average, $37 per minute to run an operating room.[4] Dedicated teams do everything faster, from starting the first case of the day with fewer delays, to cleaning and preparing rooms for the next case in 10 percent less time.[5]

Each time Matt spoke up about the issue, no matter how respectfully or collaboratively, administrators shut him down with a different excuse — if staff developed specialized knowledge, they might ask for higher pay; if they scheduled staff as teams, it would be harder to pull people for last-minute assignments that needed coverage elsewhere; what would those specialized teams do on the days the shoulder surgeons didn't operate? As a clinician, Matt was a profit-generating unit. Though he had a clear aptitude for business, administrators didn't want him spending time thinking about how to improve the system. In time, he realized that because he was an MD, and especially one without an MBA, Penn would never take his ideas seriously.

By 2006, Matt had come around to the idea that he had to find work somewhere that would honor his promise to his patients, even though such a move would put everything he'd worked for, and that he and his family had sacrificed for, on the line.

The University of Pennsylvania is a cornerstone of American medicine. Founded in 1751 by Dr. Thomas Bond and Benjamin Franklin "to care for the sick-poor and insane who were wandering the streets of Philadelphia,"[6] Pennsylvania Hospital, today part of the University of Pennsylvania health system, was the nation's first hospital. The

University of Pennsylvania opened America's first medical school fourteen years later, and the first teaching hospital, a similarly named but separate facility, the Hospital of the University of Pennsylvania, in 1874.

Just over one hundred years later, in 1993, CEO William N. Kelley, MD, decided that the only way for the Hospital of the University of Pennsylvania to remain relevant amid rapid consolidation in the regional healthcare market, like the University of Pittsburgh Medical Center from chapter 2, was to grow. He formed the University of Pennsylvania Health System, known as Penn Medicine, and over the next six years bought 270 primary care practices, acquired three hospitals, and invested in improving existing ones. To justify such explosive growth, Kelley was counting on new contracts with insurers designating Penn their preferred provider, so the patients in those 270 primary care practices would see specialists within the Penn system. And for a while, it looked like Kelley's strategy was going to pay off: In 1994 and 1995 the Hospital of the University of Pennsylvania, the health system flagship, was the most profitable hospital in the state.

Matt expected to partner with administrators when facing difficult decisions about how to allocate resources for his service. Patient care was his top priority, and he assumed his institution would feel the same way. But whenever he proposed changes, he ran into layer after layer of bureaucracy. He knew that large organizations like Penn needed bureaucracy to facilitate operations — in theory, to better help him do his job. So why did it feel like the bureaucracy and associated administrators were always working against him?

As Max Weber wrote more than a hundred years ago, bureaucracies tend to grow exponentially. At Penn, this process was accelerated by the massive expansion of the health system under Dean Kelley and by a steep increase in regulation in the 1980s and 1990s. Two pieces of legislation in particular — the Prospective Payment System in 1983, which changed Medicare reimbursement rules, and the Health Insurance Accountability and Portability Act in 1996, meant to ensure privacy and accessibility of medical records — added significant compliance and reporting burdens, and the hiring of administrators to manage them. From 1975 to 1990, the number of administrative personnel in hospitals grew 2,000 percent.[7]

The average-sized community hospital, with 161 beds and sixty-five physicians, must comply with 629 separate regulatory requirements from just four of the dozens of agencies that have a stake in hospital operations: the Centers for Medicare and Medicaid Services, the Office of the Inspector General, the Office for Civil Rights, and the Office of the National Coordinator for Health Information Technology. For that small hospital, staying compliant means hiring fifty-nine full-time administrative staff and spending $7.6 million per year recording for and reporting to those agencies, which adds $1,200 to each patient's bill. Systems the size of Penn are many times larger, and besides the dedicated compliance staff of almost forty people, almost every staff member is responsible for some aspect of recording or reporting for those federal agencies, from billing compliance auditors to medical records administrators ensuring privacy, to clinical staff doing data entry. It is telling that the chart developed to try to encapsulate the US healthcare system in 2008 put the secretary of health and human services at the center, not the patient. Patients were at the bottom right of the chart and physicians on the bottom left, separated by a sea of bureaucracy.[8]

On average, eight layers of management stand between front-line workers and the executive decision makers at healthcare behemoths like Penn, which means eight people have the authority to shut down requests for change or to flag doctors as troublemakers.[9] But when patients have a bad outcome because of those poor decisions, although lawyers often name both the doctor and the hospital in the lawsuit, doctors are an easier target. They are most proximate to the harm, do not have lawyers on staff to protect them, and may be contractually less able to mount a robust defense, due to the terms of their malpractice coverage.[10] Responsibility and accountability without authority is well known in the business world as a recipe for dysfunction and deep dissatisfaction in the workplace.[11] But in healthcare, it has become accepted practice, and the consequence for doctors like Matt, who try and fail to change their health systems, is moral injury.

Not long after Matt arrived at Penn, the capitated contracts Dean Kelley was counting on failed to materialize, as employers, facing backlash from the employees who objected to being told which physicians they could see, moved away from managed care. Falling primary care reimbursement rates also undermined Kelley's strategy of directly employing so many primary care physicians. But Kelley didn't heed early indicators of the shift away from managed care and forged ahead with his initial vision. In 1998, the system lost $98 million; in 1999, it lost $198 million. Because Penn Medicine was still tied to the University of Pennsylvania, its financial volatility threatened to bring the whole university down.

About the same time period, the health system was hit with unexpected losses. In 1995, Penn Medicine paid $30 million to settle an allegation of improper Medicare billing for physician services.[12] And in 1999, the university's research reputation had a serious setback when an eighteen-year-old volunteer underwent gene therapy for a mild condition and died days later. Though Penn only paid $517,496 in fines for the tragic outcome, broader allegations of research misconduct, conflict of interest, and a poor consent process had a lasting impact on the reputation of the institution.

In February 2000, Penn Medicine was in dire financial straits, and the university president removed Dean Kelley. After hiring a new CEO and laying off 20 percent of the workforce, the healthcare system was finally in the black in 2001. But the crisis of 1999 and 2000 cast a long shadow; austerity would determine the approach to staffing and support for years to come.[13]

It is no surprise that Jerry and Matt felt pressure to do more with less and met resistance to changes they proposed. Penn Medicine had narrowly avoided bankruptcy and now administrators were determined to follow every dime, even if that meant blowing up their relationship with a world-renowned surgeon like Jerry.

Because he was terminated so abruptly, Jerry left Penn before he'd negotiated another contract or completed the protracted credentialing process elsewhere, which is why I couldn't find any information about him at any other practices. About the time I met Matt, Jerry began negotiating a position with Rothman Orthopaedic Institute, a boutique private practice with two dozen doctors, fifteen minutes across town on the west shore of the Schuylkill River and three blocks from where the Declaration of Independence was signed. Dr. Richard Rothman, known as Dick, founded the practice in 1970 with seed funding from the media mogul Walter Annenberg, in gratitude for the care Dr. Rothman provided him. Rothman's vision was to create a center of orthopedic excellence to deliver the highest-quality musculoskeletal care to the community. In 1985, Dick forged a unique agreement with Thomas Jefferson University Hospital for Rothman, a private practice, to staff the orthopedics department for Jefferson — typically, academic centers hire physicians directly. In fact, when Matt did his orthopedics residency at Jefferson in the early 1990s, he was trained by Rothman physicians, including Dick Rothman himself.

Contracting with a private practice to staff an entire department was highly unusual, but so was the quality of surgeons Dick hired, each one outstanding in their field.

He only hired surgeons who subspecialized, and he typically assessed their skills himself. As at most private practices, new hires must prove their work ethic, academic credentials, and service-mindedness before they can buy in to the organization as partners. All surgeons at Rothman participated in some form of community service — talks, athlete care at high school games, and the like.

Unusual for a private practice, Rothman also expected partners to do research and to work with industry as thought leaders in designing better tools and implants, and unlike academic centers, Rothman let its doctors claim their own intellectual property and took none of their royalties on inventions. Rothman offered these concessions both to recruit good doctors who would otherwise choose to work at universities and because the partners didn't think it was fair to claim someone's earnings in perpetuity.

Because the physician partners owned the practice and answered only to themselves, they could choose how Rothman responded to market pressures and financial challenges, informed by their daily experience — ensuring patients and employees came first, for example — rather than having those priorities dictated by shareholder interests, or by management theories devoid of real-world input. By the time Jerry and Matt were negotiating their positions, Rothman's business model had proven itself. Patients from a two-hour radius around Philadelphia sought out doctors in the practice because of its reputation for clinical excellence and for treating patients well.

The practice had a dedicated shoulder service, but Dr. Rothman wanted to expand its clinical reach and to raise its academic clout. Bringing on Jerry and his partners was key to achieving both goals. Though Rothman offered enticing terms, it was still a boutique practice, and most doctors still assumed that high-quality research was impossible outside of academia. But Jerry's reputation as a scientist, as well as a clinician, was already well established, and he was willing to bet he could maintain a strong portfolio at Rothman through the association with Jefferson. Companies knew his value and he was confident they would continue turning to him for advice, developing total shoulder replacement implants, improved surgical instruments, or better surgical anchors. In February 2007, Jerry told Rothman he was in, but he held off on finalizing his contract so Matt would have leverage to "borrow" in his own negotiations. Recounting this story, Matt was incredulous at the kind of commitment Jerry showed toward a younger colleague. "Who *does* that?" he asked me.

After Jerry left, Matt served as the acting chief of the shoulder service while juggling both of their caseloads. For two months, he made one last effort to see if his position as chief gave him any more power or leeway to make changes to improve patient care — aligning incentives, more flexible scheduling, capping clinic sizes — and failed. Though he was deeply distressed at Penn's indifference to the needs of his patients, when Rothman reached out and offered him a position on their new shoulder service, Matt was torn. A decade younger than Jerry, he was still solidifying his standing as a specialty leader, and he worried that joining Rothman might mean the end of his academic career, his consulting opportunities, and his influence over the future of orthopedics. But if Penn could target a surgeon like Jerry, Matt knew it was only a matter of time before they came for him, too.

Matt spent several months weighing his options, talking repeatedly with Rothman, debating the pros and cons of a move, and strategizing the best way to exit. In June 2007, he decided to accept the position at Rothman and resigned from Penn. He quickly planned transitions for his patients and oversaw the graduation of his fellows, then joined Jerry at Rothman in July.

When Matt started at Rothman, he had to rebuild his practice from the ground up. But he was never happier than when his own sweat equity determined his fate. At Rothman, Matt was in control of almost every factor that determined the quality of patient care. He had the autonomy to set up his schedule as he saw fit to best facili-tate patient flow in his practice, so he was on time for every patient in clinic, with rare exceptions in emergencies. Knowing his clinics would end on time freed him up in the early evening for research or community service commitments, or to catch his daughter's soccer games. He could also diagnose a patient the same day they came in, since Rothman had long held a few imaging slots in the afternoon for same-day patients, having seen the value of leaving slack in the system over the long term.

Knowing he could make the changes necessary to create the opti-mal practice he'd envisioned, Matt put his head down and busted it, just as he had in medical school, residency, and at Penn, so he could make partner as soon as he was eligible. That would give him a seat at the decision-making table for the whole practice. But even before he made partner, the practice supported his advocacy for improvements in patient care.

Though Matt was a Rothman employee, he operated at Jefferson facilities, staffed by Jefferson clinicians — anesthesiologists, nurses, operating room technicians, and others. Like Penn, Jefferson struggled to keep teams consistent. Right away, Matt wanted to get Jefferson on board with dedicated teams. Unlike at Penn, where administrators dismissed his input, when Matt proposed piloting dedicated teams with a few surgeons, Jefferson leadership listened, in part because Dick Rothman wielded enormous influence with the organization, but also because Jefferson had bought into Rothman's patient-first approach, in hiring the practice to run the orthopedics department.

Within a year, Matt was regularly operating with the same team and the stress of his surgery days dropped dramatically. He trusted that everyone knew their role and communication became simpler. His focus, previously split between monitoring the team and attending to the surgery, shifted almost entirely to the patient. Surgeries were faster but his outcomes didn't suffer, and patients had a better experience — shorter waits in the preoperative area and less postoperative pain and nausea. As he predicted, patients weren't the only ones who benefited. Because he had time for more procedures, Matt generated more revenue. Doing the right thing for staff and patients literally paid off for Jefferson.

In 2008, two years into his time at Rothman, Matt made partner. Small group practices like Rothman rely on each member's broad aptitudes and interests to function smoothly. Matt had been fascinated by the intersections of policy, legislation, and business since his political science major in college. It was natural for him to look across those disciplines when considering next steps for the practice, and his partners quickly came to value that ability.

By 2009, Rothman employed forty-five surgeons and had enough patients that they wanted to open their own ambulatory surgery centers. Doing so would relieve some of the pressure on Jefferson operating rooms and allow them to control every aspect of surgical care for their patients — from preoperative testing to anesthesia care to amenities for waiting family members. In partnership with a private equity firm, Rothman acquired a breast surgery center that had closed early in the year, which it planned to renovate, and began construction on two new hospitals.

Then came passage of the Affordable Care Act at the end of 2009. At the last minute, lobbyists for big health systems, led by the American Hospital Association, secured the inclusion of Section 6001, which put a conditional moratorium on new physician-owned hospitals — they could open but couldn't accept Medicare or Medicaid payments, a death sentence — and disallowed expansion of existing facilities. Despite data that shows higher satisfaction, fewer complications, and lower Medicare costs at physician-owned facilities,[14] there were only around a hundred physician-owned surgical hospitals in the United States, and even together they were no match for powerful hospital lobbies, backed by the country's six thousand non-physician-owned institutions.

Just before the regulations went into effect, Rothman opened one new hospital and invested in a second with partners. Over the next few years, the partners adopted a "hold-steady" approach, hopeful that data about positive outcomes at such hospitals would sway legislators to amend Section 6001. Even though they couldn't accept public insurance payments, the hospitals were popular with privately insured patients, though the moratorium on expansion limited how many they could serve.

After five years of no progress, the partners decided it was time to take the issue directly to legislators, nominating Matt and several of his colleagues to represent the organization. In 2016, the group traveled to Washington, DC, to meet with congresspeople from

Pennsylvania and make their case for repealing Section 6001 of the Affordable Care Act.

Five years later, and fully a decade from the time the original legislation went into effect, the Centers for Medicare and Medicaid Services eased the moratorium on existing physician-owned hospital expansion, allowing rural facilities and those serving a large Medicaid population to expand with a waiver. The moratorium on Medicare and Medicaid payments is still in place, but the progress is worthy to Matt. Though he played a small role, every voice is essential when amassing support for change, and it is one step closer to Rothman adding capacity to its existing hospitals, serving more patients in the specialty model shown to improve outcomes and patient experience.

Three decades into his career, Matt still gets up at five o'clock every morning ready to work. He loves what he does, though his niggling uncertainty about the future of medicine has returned in the past few years. Today he is one of the more senior surgeons at Rothman, which has grown to nearly two hundred physicians. As the practice has expanded to maintain relevance and leverage in the region, some of the problems faced by every large organization are creeping in, as hard as the group is trying to prevent them. Some of their traditions, like monthly journal clubs where residents and attendings get to know each other informally, hosted in a different attending's home each time, have fallen away. There are communication glitches and scheduling challenges, but when issues arise, Matt knows the partners and administrative leaders approach them from a shared concern for putting patient care first.

Unlike corporations focused on quarterly profits, Matt thinks long-term. "The choices I've made are not a win," he reflected in our final conversation, "if I retire and the practice is gone a few years later." When Matt trains his residents at Jefferson, he is transparent, sharing the good, the bad, and the ugly of medicine, not to frighten or discourage them, but to prepare them for what they will face. In addition to clinical scenarios, he talks with them about the business of medicine — how money flows, how to read stakeholders, how to conduct themselves in business meetings, how to break down situations to get clarity themselves, and where the young physicians are at most risk, financially or legally. He hopes he's spent enough time honing the business acumen of those younger doctors to match the clinical skills he's imparted, so they can navigate safely through the uncertainty when his generation retires.

Owning part of the practice, having a voice and a vote in where the organization is headed, and in the tools and resources that affect his daily work and his patients' well-being, keeps Matt's risk of moral injury low. His goal is to preserve that option for future generations of surgeons.

To understand how Rothman facilitates an environment in which administrators and clinicians collaborate in service of their patients, I spoke with Ed Tufaro, Rothman's senior vice president for operations.

Although Ed didn't want to go into medicine himself, he was attracted to its healing mission, so he chose a healthcare-focused MBA over a concentration in a more lucrative sector. When Ed took the position at Rothman, he was eager to work in an organization governed by the physicians themselves, where he acts as a servant-leader. As Ed puts it, "Money is important, but I never want to lead with finances. If I do my job well, I'm taking care of the people who take care of the patients."

One of his first mentors encouraged him to "ditch the suits and put on scrubs," so he could better understand the unique challenges faced by the physicians he works with, and he did. Even in a senior leadership position, Ed solicits clinician feedback at every opportunity, takes it seriously, and tries to adapt processes, resources, or tools to address what he hears.

In *The Good Jobs Strategy*, Zeynep Ton showed how investing in employees and making operational choices that increase employee productivity, contribution, and motivation can produce more long-term profit for companies than typical cost-cutting strategies such as low wages, short staffing, and just-in-time scheduling.[15] Though Ton primarily wrote about industries with traditionally low wages, Rothman exemplifies many principles of her "good jobs strategy."

Ed strives to ensure supplies, personnel, and support are where they need to be when they need to be there, so clinicians can focus on patients, on research, or on their families, all of which he sees as important to a well-functioning workplace. As the organization grows, some bureaucracy is inevitable to keep care delivery consistent across widely dispersed locations. But Ed works tirelessly to maintain transparency by inviting physicians into the administrative process and soliciting their feedback. He reconsiders and revises decisions if physicians point out aspects he failed to consider — like how hard it was for physicians to be furloughed during the pandemic, stripped of any opportunity to practice, which for some is an essential expression of their identity. "Physicians should challenge us if our decisions create friction," he told me, "and I want them to feel that we have their backs."

Because of colleagues like Ed, Matt can practice medicine as he imagined he would when he first decided to go to medical school — patient-centered, unencumbered by layers of bureaucracy, with other physicians who shared his perspective, and the autonomy to make both business and clinical decisions about his care.

CHAPTER ELEVEN

Our Oath Is Nonnegotiable

The number of physicians in any specialty waxes and wanes as technology, scientific understanding, or economic pressures change demands for their skills. In the early 2000s, my husband, Shervin, chose radiology training for the physics and technology at the field's foundation, but his timing was also lucky; the field was burgeoning. Recruiters started calling nearly two years before he finished residency, trying to entice him to commit to a job with big signing bonuses and relocation packages. But after our experience in Rhode Island, when similar tactics landed me in a job with unsupportive leadership, labyrinthine politics, and a dead-end position with little authority, we were gun-shy.

Shervin's wish list was short, but it was surprisingly difficult to put all the elements together. Though he liked teaching, he wasn't interested enough in research to work in an academic center. He wanted to spend time with our young boys as they grew, have some flexibility to accommodate the unpredictable schedule of a two-physician household, and live where the cost of living was reasonable so we could afford land. He decided to look for a private practice where partners felt valued, and his colleagues would talk more about quality and patient care than about paychecks and bonuses. While a leadership position wasn't his goal, he wanted to have a voice. Most important, the practice leaders had to be business savvy and forward looking, anticipating changes rather than reacting to them. One of his attendings overheard him discussing his list and suggested he talk to a small practice in Harrisburg, Pennsylvania, called Tristán Associates. She'd trained with some of the partners and thought it would be a great match.

Tristán was founded by Dr. Theodore Tristán, whom everyone called Ted. Born in Mexico, he moved with his family to Rochester, New York, when he was a child so his father could work for Kodak. Drafted out of college, Ted served in World War II as an X-ray technician. After the war, he finished college and medical school, then served as a general medical officer during the Korean War before finally training in radiology at the University of Pennsylvania. That experience attuned him to what both patients and clinicians needed from radiologists, setting him apart in a field known for having little patient contact. He practiced in Rochester, New York, for several years, then returned to Pennsylvania in 1967 and set up a hospital-based private group practice, known as Tristán Associates, at Polyclinic Hospital in Harrisburg.

Ted had high expectations for his partners and his staff. In an article commemorating Dr. Tristán after his death in 2011, Dr. Milton Friedlander, who trained under Ted in Rochester and followed him to Harrisburg, recalled, "He used to browbeat me. He was a guy who played by the book. He was meticulous about every darned detail in life." But, Friedlander continued, "He was such an honest, decent person. I couldn't have followed a better man."[1]

Perhaps because he grew up hearing about the latest discoveries at Kodak, Ted was constantly scanning the horizon for innovations in imaging. In the late 1960s, new tests like low-dose mammography, ultrasound, and CT scans allowed doctors to visualize internal organs without exploratory surgery. As the quality of images improved, and more specialties relied on imaging to make diagnostic and treatment decisions, demand began to outstrip the capacity of hospital departments, and Ted started thinking about setting up an outpatient radiology practice. In 1974, he paired the capabilities of a hospital-like department with a low-key outpatient setting, recalling the home offices of some early radiologists, for management of less urgent cases.[2] Patients liked the convenience, physicians appreciated the more predictable schedule, and the practice quickly developed a loyal following.

In 1976, the American Cancer Society recommended yearly screening mammography for every woman over fifty. But mammograms were poorly reimbursed, so most practices viewed them as low priority, and radiologists read the studies at their own convenience. Patients might wait weeks for results only to learn that the radiologist needed more images to make a diagnosis. Ted thought subjecting women to weeks of avoidable anxiety every year was unacceptable, so he made mammograms central to the business model of his new practice. Women make 85 percent of the healthcare decisions in their families; if they were treated well, Ted was confident they would spread the word in their social circles that Tristán was the place to go for imaging needs.

Each day, a dedicated radiologist read mammograms as soon as the films were ready, while the women waited for their results. Extra views were done immediately, and they looked at any suspicious areas with ultrasound. Most of the time, women left within two hours, reassured they were free of detectable cancer and didn't need to come back for a year. If a biopsy was needed, the office scheduled it within days. By 1985, the strategy of treating mammograms as a loss leader was so successful that Ted opened the Harrisburg Breast Diagnostic Center, the first such outpatient facility in the area.

Whenever possible, the radiologists also extended this courtesy to other studies. This led to an unusual phenomenon for doctors in the specialty — patients at Tristán often knew their radiologists personally, and some even requested appointments with specific doctors. Referring doctors, too, appreciated the personalized attention they received from physicians at Tristán. They knew they would get a call from one of the radiologists if a study was worrisome, rather than waiting several days for the report, and they could trust their patients would be treated with courtesy, respect, and compassion from every level of staff — front desk to radiologist to billing office — which was rare in larger systems.

Long before Zeynep Ton coined the phrase, Tristán had created a "Good Jobs" practice: The partners paid close attention to operations by standardizing processes but empowering employees to deviate if their judgment deemed it important; operated with slack in all systems, slightly overstaffing and underscheduling to accommodate inevitable emergencies for staff or for patients who needed urgent imaging; and invested in employees by offering good salaries and benefits, sufficient training, and healthy bonuses in good years. As a result, the practice enjoyed low turnover and a solid revenue stream driven by loyal patients. By the time Shervin was talking to Tristán, they had several offices in the Harrisburg area staffed by about twenty doctors and two hundred support staff and had expanded to provide ultrasounds, CT, MRI, and PET scans.

After several phone conversations with Joe Bellissimo, the current president of the practice, and a few of the partners, we flew down to meet the group. Two days of interviews and hours of informal conversations later, we made our decision, which came down to two main factors: the leadership of the practice and the other radiologists who would be Shervin's partners.

Joe Bellissimo's genuineness, incisive wit, and charisma set the tone for the organization. He grew up in Pittsburgh when it was a struggling rust belt city, during the economic lull between the collapse of US Steel and the ascendance of the University of Pittsburgh Medical Center. Though his father, a horn player, trained at Juilliard, he couldn't make ends meet as a classical musician, so he sold encyclopedias, then industrial cleaning equipment, and eventually owned his own gas station and car wash. Joe grew up working for the family businesses, and he learned much of his business savvy and hustle from his dad.

He graduated from West Virginia University, where he met his wife, who was in pharmacy school. Then he began nearly a decade at Penn State Hershey Medical Center, first in medical school, then in residency, interrupted by two years serving in the Indian Health Service in Montana in exchange for partial forgiveness of his loans. As it had for Ted, two years of practicing primary care sensitized Joe to the need for fast, accurate test results.

Joe took the job with Tristán in 1982, straight out of his radiology residency. He chose Tristán because of Ted's integrity, but also because protected time away from medicine helped his radiologists practice at their best. Joe valued time with his family and time for his other interests — riding horses, restoring cars, renovating and building houses, and hunting big game. It was easy to see Joe and his wife, who is a powerhouse in her own right, as our future selves. They lived on a small farm with three boys, about a decade older than our two, to whom they were thoughtful, full-contact parents who balanced empathy with high expectations and a healthy dose of humor. And that's the same way Joe guided the practice, after becoming president in 1990.

The partners who would be Shervin's colleagues were serious about the practice and about maintaining their leading role in patient care in the clinical community, but their jousting banter made it clear they were also friends, and it was easy to be with them. During our visit, Dr. Mark Labuski, one of the newest partners, shared with Shervin his perspective on what set Tristán apart: "This is a group that is more interested in taking care of the community than they are taking care of themselves, but we also take care of each other."

Mark grew up in Bentley Creek, Pennsylvania, a small town with a parking lot full of Amish buggies at the grocery store on Saturday mornings. He went to medical school at Penn State on a military scholarship, did his internship with the navy, and served as a general medical officer and brigade surgeon at Camp Lejeune in Jacksonville, North Carolina, for three years before returning to Penn State for a radiology residency, where he was chief resident in his final year.

Tristán had offered jobs to almost every chief resident at Penn State prior to Mark, but when he graduated in 2000, the practice was ending its decadeslong inpatient radiology contract with Polyclinic to focus on outpatient imaging, and they weren't ready to hire another physician. Although Mark took a job at a small hospital in Huntingdon, Pennsylvania, he and Joe stayed in touch. Three years later, Tristán had work for him, and a long-term plan. Joe had another ten years before he planned to retire, and he knew it would take the better part of that time to train his successor. Mark had risen to leadership positions almost everywhere he'd been and had worked in central Pennsylvania long enough to have a handle on local healthcare politics. Joe was confident Mark had the aptitude to lead the practice, and he hoped with enough coaching and encouragement, Mark would also express interest in stepping up.

We left the visit infatuated with the practice and captivated by Pennsylvania. Shervin signed a contract in the summer of 2004 then finished out his residency and a year of fellowship. We bought our farm in the fall of 2005, said a year of sad, slow good-byes to the Upper Valley of New Hampshire, and moved from our quarter-acre in-town lot to thirteen acres in Carlisle, a thirty-minute drive from Harrisburg, in late June 2006, ready for a very different life.

Shervin was born in 1967 in Tehran, Iran, twelve years before the Iranian Revolution ousted Mohammad Reza Shah Pahlavi and replaced the monarchy with an Islamic republic. His father, Ru, grew up in Tehran, left school at thirteen, and embarked on a lifetime of serial entrepreneurship, always looking for his next big win. His mother, Parvin, was the eldest of thirteen children from Kerman, a cold desert city of half a million people along Saheb Al Zaman Mountain in south-central Iran. She never finished high school, but in her mid-twenties she moved to Tehran to study fashion. She became fast friends with a fellow student, Nina, who introduced Parvin to her brother Ru. A year later, in July 1966, Ru and Parvin married; the next summer, Shervin was born.

At Ru's urging, Parvin struck out on her own after fashion school, opening a bespoke clothing boutique in a trendy neighborhood in

northern Tehran popular with American oil executives and their
wives. Parvin and Ru befriended one such couple, and in 1974 they
helped Ru establish himself in Dallas as Iran began inching toward
revolution. Parvin and Shervin joined him in 1975. Four years later,
when the Shah was deposed, Parvin and Ru were cut off from their
family back in Iran.

In Dallas, Ru's demeanor was tumultuous at best, and the marriage
broke under the strain when Shervin was eleven. Parvin, on the other
hand, was as consistent as Ru was chaotic. Her first job in America
was in the alterations department at the original Neiman Marcus store
in downtown Dallas, and she spent her career with the company,
eventually working her way up to director of alterations for the southwest region. By the time she retired, she was the national alterations
department troubleshooter, who still did high-stakes alterations on
haute couture gowns other tailors were afraid to touch.

Early on, Shervin was fascinated by the brain and by literature, but he
reasoned it would be possible to still appreciate literature as a doctor and
impossible to do the reverse. Intent on becoming a neurosurgeon, he
double-majored in English literature and biology at Cornell University.
Confident he would get in everywhere, Shervin applied to only a handful
of medical schools and was shocked to find himself rejected everywhere
except at Cornell and the University of Texas at Houston, where he was
wait-listed. Days before classes were to start in August, UT Houston
took him off the waiting list. Once in medical school, the sheer volume
of material taxed his intellect for the first time. His classmates were every
bit as smart as he was, and many were accustomed to studying much
harder. Though four years in medical school humbled Shervin, he still
did well enough to match into the single neurosurgery residency slot
available each year at Dartmouth. In 1993, he started his intern year as I
started my third year of my surgical residency.

The surgery department was small, with about fifty residents,
across all specialties, in the hospital one hundred hours each week,
constantly bumping into one another in the emergency room, in

operating rooms, in radiology, and in the call suite. During our few hours off each week, many of us also socialized together. Shervin and I had our first accidental date at a dive bar in downtown Hanover the Monday after Thanksgiving when no one else showed up to watch *Monday Night Football*.

We were engaged by March, and weeks later I resigned from my surgery residency. That summer, Shervin began his first year of neuro-surgery rotations while I worked in rural emergency rooms and coor-dinated our fall wedding. Although he loved the diagnostic challenges and felt at home in the operating room, by the spring of his second year, he decided he couldn't spend his career watching brain tumors, ruptured aneurysms, or spinal cord injuries ravage his patients with-out being able to cure very many of them. He, too, resigned from his residency and started working emergency room shifts. Five years later, Shervin realized what he loved most about surgery and emer-gency medicine was the imaging, and he returned to Dartmouth for a radiology residency. His playfulness and unguarded joy, which I'd fallen in love with and watched slip away during his neurosurgery year, returned when he restarted in the residency that was right for him. As hard as it was to be back in the grind of training, it was worth it knowing he'd found his specialty.

Shervin was drawn to radiology because it is one of the most consis-tently progressive fields in medicine. Advanced imaging — CT, MRI, and PET scans — emerged into widespread use roughly forty years ago, and more powerful computing consistently improved the accu-racy of these images. Every specialty has benefited: Orthopedists visualize complex injuries and plan surgery before operating, cranio-facial surgeons build precise guides for reconstructing delicate facial structures, oncologists track the progress of cancer treatments, and obstetricians show parents their child's face months before birth. But radiologic studies are also expensive, and payers have long debated whether they are used appropriately.

Radiologic studies are done in three settings: hospitals, including their outpatient departments; outpatient radiology offices that perform a variety of tests, like X-rays, CT, MRI, PET, and ultrasounds; and non-radiology outpatient offices that typically offer one or two types of imaging, ostensibly for patient convenience but also to generate revenue for those practices. In the early 2000s, several factors led to a rapid rise in imaging in all types of settings: better technology, such as new, less invasive, yet still fast and accurate studies that allowed diagnosis of conditions such as heart vessel blockages or colon cancer; patient requests driven by online research; and physicians who, increasingly pressed for time, found it quicker and easier to order imaging than to convince patients they didn't need it, or to do a careful history and physical. The increase in imaging orders was particularly steep at non-radiology outpatient practices. Multiple studies found that non-radiology physicians who owned their own equipment, and earned revenue from it, ordered imaging more often — sometimes as much as seven times more frequently — than those who referred to a radiologist.[3]

The Deficit Reduction Act of 2005 took aim at those self-referrals. To reduce the federal deficit, bloated by military spending on the wars in Iraq and Afghanistan, the act cut federal spending by $39 billion, including $11 billion from Medicare. Late in the negotiations, legislation targeting $3 billion in Medicare funding for radiologic studies was slipped into the bill, without public hearing, a comment period, or feedback from stakeholders.[4] The language failed to distinguish between non-radiology, self-referred outpatient imaging venues and radiology-run practices, which had not been identified as a cause of increased spending. All outpatient practices that provided imaging would see reduced reimbursement for 65 percent of imaging studies for Medicare patients.[5]

Tristán fought for amended language for two years before the cuts went into effect, writing letters, talking with state and national legislators about the unintended consequences to independent outpatient radiology practices, and supporting actions by the American College of Radiology, to no avail. On January 1, 2007, six months into Shervin's new job, the reimbursement cuts to outpatient radiology went into effect. Overnight, revenue to the practice fell by half. Because Tristán provided no services that might offset the losses, the only way for the practice to survive was to slash payroll. To spare the support staff and new hires, the partners took deep cuts to their own salaries, making less than half what they had the previous year.

Many evenings, after we put our boys to bed, Shervin and I had difficult conversations about the tenuousness of his position. We thought he had found a place he could spend his career, and suddenly everything was in flux again, though now we had far fewer options. In the wake of the legislation, demand for radiologists, especially outpatient positions, had dried up; if Tristán went under, finding another similar job would be difficult. We were loath to uproot our boys and leave our farm, but neither of us relished Shervin returning to inpatient work, with shifts to cover around the clock, every day of the year. But as much as I worried, Shervin did not. He was confident in his role at Tristán, having already made himself indispensable to the practice for his knowledge, technical skills, and productivity. More important, he trusted Joe would get them out of this scrape.

In the end, the practice couldn't avoid laying off support staff and technicians — something they had never done before. To the partners, it felt like turning family out in the cold, but they agreed they had no choice. Joe also took on contracts for work at far-flung hospitals, some as much as two hours from Harrisburg. Though these actions saved the practice, Tristán was left teetering on the edge of its business model. All the clinicians were doing more work with less support, and cutting any further might impact the care they provided to patients.

Then the recession of 2008 hit, and healthcare, like every other sector of the economy, suffered. Millions of people ended up unemployed and uninsured. Those who still had jobs worried they might soon lose them and were reluctant to get testing that wasn't critical. At

Tristán, patient volumes fell, and revenue dropped below subsistence levels. If they didn't find a solution, the practice might not survive.

In January 2009, Shervin became a partner and began attending the monthly board meetings. Each partner had some notable quirk — the inveterate clotheshorse and former blackjack dealer; the occasionally imperious, always stylish Iraqi; the curmudgeonly retired military officer with an encyclopedic knowledge of whiskey — that was in turns trying and endearing. As heated as their debates could get, though — and some were especially tense in this period of even tighter revenue contraction — they always parted as family at the end of the meetings.

One of Shervin's first votes as partner was in favor of Mark Labuski as vice president of the practice. He knew Mark was a servant-leader who would choose the good of their patients, and the practice as a whole, over his own personal interests. In his observation, Mark was as comfortable and respectful talking to a chief executive as he was to frightened and uncomfortable patients during procedures. During the most challenging discussions, he had a way of settling the room by breaking vexing issues into their essential elements and tackling them one at a time.

That same evening, Joe shared some very bad news: Because of the recession, the financial situation of the practice had grown even more precarious. In his estimation, Tristán was now unsustainable as an independent group. Subsequent partner meetings became hours-long marathons of financial reviews and strategy debates. Some of those nights, Shervin wasn't home until after midnight and was too troubled by the discussions to rehash them until days later. Now he was as worried as I was — about the future of the practice and of his field and whether we might lose the life we'd worked so hard to build.

With Mark learning at his right hand, Joe explored every possible option to keep Tristán viable. He considered mergers with other practices and strategic partnerships, in the meantime taking on more contracts just to stay afloat, which stretched all the physicians very thin. Whenever there was a major decision to make, the partners would debate whether a given option would allow them to implement their practice model. At one point, Shervin recounted Joe Bellissimo saying that if the radiologists couldn't provide timely, relevant care to patients, nothing else mattered. Only when they were assured of that did they focus on their other priorities: whether they could pay their bills and take time off. For two years, the partners voted down every option Joe presented. No amount of money could convince them to compromise how they practiced.

Finally, Joe negotiated a deal with Mike Young, the CEO of Pinnacle Health, the same regional health system that briefly employed Hannah Becker from chapter 2, for Tristán to sell its offices and equipment to Pinnacle and become a contract group, with the radiologists providing physician services to the Pinnacle locations they used to own. Pinnacle would own the facilities and machines and would control the scheduling of technicians and staff, who were now their employees, instead of Tristán's. Both parties agreed that Tristán would see an increase in patient volume when Pinnacle physicians could make in-network referrals to Tristán radiologists.

Fair compensation for the radiologists depended on that flow of patients, though, and the whole deal depended on an uneasy truce with a long-standing competitor, Quantum, which staffed Pinnacle's inpatient services and the non-Tristán outpatient locations. Quantum leadership had a reputation for being unapologetically business-oriented to the point of ruthlessness; in informal conversations with one of Shervin's partners, former employees described productivity trackers that spun like odometers on their workstations and cameras monitoring their activities.

Despite their reservations, the partners all agreed the deal was the best possible option. On Monday, March 12, 2012, the contract with Pinnacle officially started. Though Joe planned to remain with Tristán for at least another five years, he wanted to facilitate a smooth transition of power, so at the next board meeting, he stepped down as president, and the group unanimously elected Mark their new leader.

While the partners expected some bumps in the transition from controlling their own practice to working within a much larger system, no one imagined how precarious their situation would soon become.

The first two years with Pinnacle were smooth, if a bit slower than Tristán expected. Then in 2014, Pinnacle and Penn State Hershey Medical Center signed a letter of intent for a proposed merger. Such a letter triggers a review by the Federal Trade Commission for any potential restraint of competition. While that review was under way, the three radiology groups — Tristán, Quantum, and Penn State — began discussions about how they would integrate their services once the organizations merged. With three different cultures, workflows, scheduling, and staffing models to align, there was a lot to work out, and the conversations stalled. Shervin got the impression, from Mark's reports, that the leaders of one of the other groups would fully participate only after the merger went through.

While the merger was under review, Tristán patient volume was in free fall. Their chief financial officer had a keen eye for trends, and he'd never been so far off in his predictions. It would be one thing, Shervin remarked to me, if volume dropped across the board. But while Tristán's volume was falling, the rest of Pinnacle's numbers looked good. Mark asked Pinnacle administration for insight and got nowhere.

Eventually, information started to trickle back to Tristán about potential reasons for this discrepancy. After one especially maddening partner meeting, Shervin came home livid. One partner shared that his wife had tried to schedule an appointment at a Tristán office, but the Pinnacle scheduler told her Tristán offices had no availability. She knew from her husband that wasn't true, but the scheduler refused to offer those locations.

From conversations with radiologists at Penn State, Mark knew there would be plenty of additional work for them as soon as the merger went through, but Tristán couldn't wait that long. Mark approached Mike Young about amending their exclusive contract so Tristán could supplement their income with work elsewhere. When they spoke, Mark confronted Mike about his role in issues like low patient volume, and by the end of the conversation, Mike agreed to let Tristán radiologists start covering overflow for Penn State right away.

Then, in October 2016, a federal appeals court ruled in favor of the Federal Trade Commission, and Penn State's board of directors announced their decision to drop the proposed merger. "The merger would have likely led to lower quality and higher cost healthcare," said a representative from the Federal Trade Commission, "at the expense of Harrisburg residents and their employers."[6] Shervin came home dejected after the board meeting following that announcement. Three senior staff — two partners and the chief financial officer — had announced they would be retiring in December. Though all of them had hoped to work a few more years, they didn't want to keep drawing salaries the organization could not afford. One of those partners was Joe Bellissimo, and it felt like the end of an era.

Shortly after that meeting, Shervin lost his appetite and grew increasingly short of breath. An arrhythmia was interfering with his heart's function, and fluid was slowly building up in his lungs and abdomen. Throughout the late fall and early winter, Pinnacle cardiologists tried, unsuccessfully, to get control of his condition. Meanwhile, his partners, no questions asked, stepped in for him whenever he had an appointment, or switched assignments with him when he didn't feel up to a long commute. The night the air ambulance couldn't fly, Joe Bellissimo even called Mike Young to pressure him into transferring Shervin immediately, rather than waiting until the next morning. Shervin stayed home until late February, and he never worried about covering his shifts or whether he would still have a job when he recovered.

In August 2017, the University of Pittsburgh Medical Center bought Pinnacle, and Tristán's contract with it. UPMC was notorious for imposing its own practice models on acquired physicians, and we all worried Tristán was on the brink of collapse. Shortly thereafter, two of the younger partners, who weren't yet deeply committed to central Pennsylvania, left for other positions. But for our ties to the community, we might have done the same, and no one at Tristán would have blamed us.

Then, in December 2017, the first glimmer of a good opportunity appeared when Penn State and Highmark Blue Cross Blue Shield, a regional insurer, announced a strategic partnership to develop the Community Medical Group, a network of community medical offices affiliated with the academic medical center. Each physician leader, no matter which department or group, would be paired with an administrator, which meant clinicians, who know best what's required for patient care, would again have real decision-making power. This "dyad model of management" in healthcare dates back to 1908 when William May hired Harry Harwick to manage the growing operations at the newly formed Mayo Clinic. In recent years, healthcare systems have revived the concept, recognizing that administrators and clinicians both bring unique and essential expertise to decision making.

The physician leader behind the initiative, Dr. William Bird, viewed radiology services as the crucial element in the new endeavor. "Because radiology touches nearly every patient and disease category . . . it becomes clear that the influence of radiology on the cost and quality of care across the entire system is even larger than profit statistics suggest."[7] Beyond the finances, Dr. Bird hoped that Tristán's model of patient-first care would influence the other departments in the Community Medical Group.

Mark was keen to begin negotiations with Penn State, but there was a problem: The contract with UPMC included a restrictive covenant preventing physicians from taking jobs with competing organizations within thirty miles of UPMC locations, which blanketed central and western Pennsylvania. For months, the partners waited while Mark explored how they might move forward. Finally, in July 2018, Shervin got a call from Mark while we were on vacation at our house in the Ozarks. "They let us out!" he exclaimed from across the porch. "I don't know how Mark did it, but they let us go. No thirty miles, no years to wait. We can talk to Penn State tomorrow!" His relief was palpable, and we celebrated with margaritas at the local Mexican restaurant that night.

Though the Community Medical Group seemed an ideal arrangement, the experience with Pinnacle had left many partners understandably wary. But wary or not, they had to make a move. Mark began negotiations, which progressed rapidly, and within a few months, it was time for a final vote. Partnering with Penn State would mean dissolving the practice and becoming direct employees of the Community Medical Group. Some of the partners were troubled by the prospect of losing the institution that had anchored their professional lives and by what felt like a betrayal of Ted Tristán, who had made it possible for them to practice in alignment with their values. In preparation for the final board meeting, Joe counseled some of the physicians who'd been with the practice longest: "For Ted, what mattered was the culture. If we can move the group to Penn State and keep the culture the same, while taking care of our patients, Ted would be happy." They voted unanimously to adapt the structure of their practice, rather than compromise their values.

On Sunday, December 31, 2018, Tristán Radiology Associates disbanded, and on Tuesday, January 2, 2019, the twelve remaining partners began work as Penn State Community Medical Group employees.

Three years into the agreement with Penn State, I can see the relief in Shervin's face. He never complained about Pinnacle, but he looks forward to going to work again. Tristán physicians designed the scheduling, workflow, and staffing structure for the community radiology sites, so they have control of important and often-overlooked details, like leaving slack in the system, including three reserved slots every day for urgent appointments. As needed, they select new equipment and work together to hire new radiologists to meet increasing demands. Mark works closely with Tim Mosher, his counterpart in the flagship hospital's academic radiology group, to keep their departments aligned, and they both maintain a clinical practice so they are "player-coaches," much like the Rothman physicians in the previous chapter. Each also works hand-in-glove with an administrative counterpart whose mandate is to facilitate good clinical care.

The difference is playing out daily. While I was writing this chapter, a friend texted me in a panic. The year before, Lori's mammogram at another system was abnormal, and the radiology group wanted her to wait a month for additional views. Her husband, who is a physician in that system, found a slot in the schedule for her two days later. But he also voiced his frustrations to administrators, who assured him that next time there would be no delays. A year later, my friend had another abnormal study, and the same radiology group scheduled her for additional views in two weeks. Exasperated, my friend called Shervin.

Because the radiology office at the Community Medical Group had slots reserved for same-day appointments, they could fit her in within hours. The billing office representative, who has been with Tristán for decades, ran her insurance to make sure she wouldn't sustain a big financial hit for visiting an out-of-network provider, or for having two studies on the same day. The scheduler conveyed the financial information to Lori and gave her instructions for how to obtain the images that had been done at the other facility earlier that day and the previous year, so the radiologist could compare them all. At her appointment, Lori answered screening questions about her ancestry she'd never heard before, which would enable the radiologists to calculate her risk of future malignancy and recommend more frequent or more targeted testing accordingly. The technician then took additional views and did an ultrasound, and the physician confirmed the findings immediately. She left an hour later with the diagnosis of a harmless condition, relieved and grateful for the experience of being well cared for every step of the way. Her husband, a doctor rendered helpless by his own system earlier in the day, felt like Tristán cared for him, too. It was a tremendous relief to feel the collegiality that had been missing for too long.

There are still challenges on the horizon, each of which is testing Tristán's commitment to its practice model that minimizes the risk of moral injury. Reimbursement structures, driven by Medicare legislation, are constantly in flux. William Bird, the champion of the Community Medical Group and a strong proponent of Tristán's approach, recently retired; new leadership means change, and not always for the better. Finally, because the practice has been successful, it's growing, with the attendant challenge of maintaining their high clinical standards and their patient-centered, service-minded culture.

But the members of Tristán will face those challenges as they faced others, by reaffirming their shared value of delivering the highest-quality patient care in every decision; by being willing to make intense, short-term personal sacrifices for the long-term good of the practice; by showing deep respect and caring for one another, and for everyone with whom they work; and by focusing more on doing good than on doing well. No matter the practice environment, they measure their success according to whether they have stayed true to Ted Tristán's original vision to "serve the patient, first and foremost, but also serve the clinician."

CHAPTER TWELVE

Showdown

When Ray Brovont picked up the phone at 6:30 A.M. on a sticky Kansas morning in the summer of 2016, he knew it was probably bad news. Shifts were about to change in the emergency room at Overland Park Regional Medical Center, where he had been the medical director for nearly four years; if one of his staff was calling him at home, it was because there was something he needed to know before he got to work, so he could prepare himself to manage the fallout.

"Ray, I feel like this is my fault," his colleague, who I'll call Dr. Eric Sosa, began, "but I don't know what else I could have done. Can you help me think it through?" Eric recounted what had transpired during his overnight shift in a flood of staccato phrases, his mind running faster than his words could follow, anxious for absolution.

An overhead page just after midnight sent Eric, the only doctor in the hospital assigned to cover emergencies, dashing upstairs to the intensive care unit to respond to a "Code Blue" for a patient who had stopped breathing. Mindful that he couldn't leave the emergency room uncovered for long, he resuscitated and stabilized the patient as quickly as he could. After making sure the nurses had all the orders they needed and calling the patient's physician and family, he returned to the emergency room.

As Eric walked in, he heard the patient in Room 2 groaning softly and saw him twist from side to side on the narrow gurney. Grabbing the chart, he saw they had been waiting for forty-five minutes, and one glance at the cardiac tracing showed Eric the patient was having a major heart attack. He called the nurse over, alarmed, and initiated the chest pain protocol. Eric saw the automatic reading suggested a heart attack; he also knew they were unreliable — confirming a heart attack required a doctor's interpretation — but if there was even a chance the reading was correct, why hadn't anyone paged him or called the intensive care unit?

Even if he had been paged, Eric would still have stayed to resuscitate the patient in intensive care who was not breathing. But he would have waited to call that patient's physician and family until he had mobilized the cardiac catheterization teams for the patient with chest pain. Every minute of delay means more muscle cells die, increasing the risk of permanent damage or death. The American Heart Association's guidelines gave him ninety minutes, at most, to diagnose a heart attack and for a colleague to insert an artery-opening stent.

With a patient in trouble, Eric didn't have time to waste wondering why he hadn't been called. He kicked the department into high gear, mobilizing the cardiology team, administering drugs to relieve the patient's pain and to try to get more blood flow to his heart, and preparing the patient for surgery. Though he got the patient to the catheterization suite as quickly as he could, and the cardiologists opened the artery with a stent, the whole process, including the time the patient spent waiting to be examined, took more than two hours.

Ray, who was equally mystified as to why Eric had not been called — maybe the nurses didn't want to distract him during the code and knew he'd be back as soon as he could — reassured him there was nothing he could have done differently. Before they got off the phone, he offered the consolation that, confronted with an actual tragedy rather than a theoretical possibility, their administrators would surely have no choice but to increase emergency room staffing and change the Code Blue policy.

As soon as he became medical director in 2012, Ray began warning leadership at EmCare that staffing the emergency room with only one physician for eighteen hours each day and making that doctor responsible for inpatient emergencies in another part of the hospital was putting patients at risk. When the hospital expanded in 2014, doubling the number of emergency beds and increasing inpatient beds by more than 50 percent, without a corresponding increase in staffing, the situation became even more precarious.

When Overland Park opened a ten-bed pediatric emergency room in 2016, hospital administration and EmCare leadership agreed that from 11:00 P.M. to 11:00 A.M., the pediatric emergency room would not be staffed by a dedicated pediatric emergency physician. Over Ray's objections, EmCare held one emergency physician responsible for all adult emergency patients, all after-hours pediatric patients, and inpatient Code Blue calls. They might be needed in three places at once.

Less than an hour after he hung up the phone with Eric, Ray got into work and checked in with the cardiologists. The patient's condition was touch and go, as it remained for the next two days. On the third morning, he learned the patient had died in the night.

Ray was livid. Though his staff had done their best, a patient had suffered because of constraints beyond their control. This was not the care they had pledged to provide when they went into medicine. Determined this would never happen at his hospital again, Ray intensified his campaign to leadership to increase emergency room staffing to appropriate levels.

Speaking up about patient safety got him fired, so Ray sued EmCare for wrongful termination. Litigation dragged on for more than four years, until 2021, when a Missouri court of appeals upheld a $26 million award in his favor. Such a large judgment against two massive healthcare corporations was shocking enough, but what held my attention when I saw the news were the details of the case itself, which read like a how-to manual for physicians to use in fighting back against an employer setting them up for moral injury.[1]

Since publishing our first article in *STAT News*, physicians facing moral injury had been contacting me almost every day, but most were unprepared or unwilling to speak publicly about their distress because they feared retaliation. In 2020, two doctors in Mississippi and one in

Washington State had been fired after advocating for stronger safety measures in their hospitals at the start of the pandemic.[2] Two major studies, one in 1998 and a follow-up in 2013, confirmed that physicians knew they could be fired with little or no reason and without due process.[3] Many institutions warn their staff that speaking to the press could result in disciplinary action, including termination.[4] As a result, most doctors, even those who are deeply distressed, suffer in silence. But not Ray Brovont.

I was eager to know why Ray was different, so I found his email address and reached out. He wrote back right away, and we had several long conversations in the ensuing year about his background, how his case unfolded, what prepared him to take on this fight, and what others could learn from his actions.

Ray grew up in Livermore, California, a small city on the eastern edge of the San Francisco Bay Area. As a child, he wanted to be an engineer, but feeling helpless after his grandfather had a stroke changed his mind, and he latched on to the "organic engineering" of medicine to satisfy his powerful drive to heal others.

When he was in high school, his parents divorced, and the related financial strain left little to fund college for Ray and his two sisters. His father and grandfather, both navy veterans, encouraged him to consider joining the military to pay for his studies. Heeding their advice, Ray attended the University of California–Davis on a full scholarship from the Reserve Officer Training Corps, or ROTC. After earning a degree in biology, he began medical school at George Washington University, on a merit-based scholarship, in 1997.

In July 2001, Ray moved to Fort Hood, Texas, for his emergency medicine residency. At the end of August, he married his wife, a lawyer with a master of public health degree whom he met when they were both at George Washington, and they returned from their brief honeymoon just days before the United States was forever changed on September 11.

Like Rita Gallardo from chapter 7, rather than support a peace-time force, Ray would spend his military service caring for troops at war as a result of the terrorist attacks. After finishing his residency in 2004, he was stationed at Winn Army Hospital in Georgia. In 2005, Ray deployed to Iraq for thirteen months, where he served as brigade surgeon, responsible for the care of up to six thousand troops and the medical initiatives implemented by that unit. His understanding of infantry operations, thanks to his ROTC background, helped him craft effective medic training in battlefield medicine. Speaking the language of "the line" gave him added credibility with non-medical officers, who paid close attention to his recommendations. In his role, Ray also worked with the Iraqi army, police, and national guard to train local emergency medical technicians to provide advanced care during trans-port to a hospital and to staff a community clinic. He relished knowing that patients received excellent care from those he trained and led.

When Ray left the military in 2008 after seven years of service, he and his wife settled in her hometown of Kansas City, Kansas. He took a job with EmCare, the largest hospital staffing company in the United States and the same corporation that provided emergency department services to Carlisle Regional Medical Center in chapter 2. Every hospital checks the credentials of each doctor who works in the facility, whether employed directly or as a contractor, a process that takes months and requires reams of paperwork. EmCare streamlined parts of the credentialing process, so it was easier for Ray to fill shifts at several hospitals, on either side of the state line — he held licenses in both Kansas and Missouri — without doing additional paperwork. He expected that a large, successful healthcare corporation would maintain high quality standards and adhere to national guidelines, regulations, and legislation, all of which aligned with his own values. If he succeeded, he hoped advancement in the organization would follow as it had in the army.

His first assignment from EmCare was in the emergency depart-ment at Centerpoint Medical Center, a 257-bed community hospital

owned by the Hospital Corporation of America, HCA, and located in
Independence, Missouri, just east of Kansas City, Missouri, and home
of the thirty-third US president, Harry Truman. Like most other small
hospitals, Centerpoint struggled to attract board-certified emergency
physicians, who shy away from remote, resource-constrained settings
that are so different from the urban hospitals where most of them
trained. Several years earlier, the hospital started paying EmCare a
fixed annual fee to recruit, retain, and schedule emergency physicians.
EmCare also handled billing insurers and patients for the services
their physicians provided, and sometimes shared a portion of that
revenue with the hospital.

At Centerpoint, Ray consistently had some of the highest patient
satisfaction scores of all the doctors on staff. He regularly exceeded
performance targets, like how many patients he saw each hour, how
long wait times were when he worked, and how quickly he moved
patients out of the emergency room, either back to their homes or
to an inpatient bed at the hospital. Other staff in the department
requested to work with him; he was competent, collegial, and inspired
confidence.

In 2012, EmCare asked him to be the medical director of the emergency room at Overland Park Regional Medical Center, in Overland
Park, Kansas, fifteen minutes southwest of downtown Kansas City.
Eager to put his operational and leadership skills to use, Ray immediately accepted.

Like Centerpoint, Overland Park was part of the massive HCA
health system and had relied on EmCare to staff the emergency room
for several years. A few months before Ray started at Overland Park,
HCA and EmCare entered what is known as a joint venture. Whereas
the companies were previously separate parties in a contracted relationship, they would now share ownership of the staffing arrangement. But Ray wasn't intimidated by the prospect of navigating that
big bureaucracy, nor by long chains of command; he'd spent years in
the army training to work in just that kind of environment.

At Overland Park, Ray set out to re-create the culture of collegiality, support, and operational excellence he'd learned in the army. Under his leadership, Overland Park's emergency room became extremely efficient. The department had the best patient satisfaction scores of any emergency room in the region, and other performance indicators were enviable: average wait times of six minutes compared with a national average of sixty minutes; door-to-pain-control time of 15 minutes when many hospitals took more than an hour; door-to-admission time of 167 minutes compared with a national average of 247.[5] Within a year of starting at Overland Park, it wasn't just clinicians in his hospital who wanted to work with his team; Ray had a waiting list of nurses and physicians at other area hospitals who wanted to transfer to his facility, and he'd earned a reputation for working across divisions to make changes in the best interest of both his patients and colleagues.

Ray's team in the emergency room touched virtually every other sector in the hospital, and he encouraged them to solve the problems they encountered, because pooling expertise led to the best patient care. One of the first issues he tackled was pain control. Hospital policy, shaped by hospital lawyers, dictated that the orders emergency room physicians wrote to admit patients expired after eight hours. Physicians on call in the inpatient units often had to reassess patients in the middle of the night, though their new orders rarely changed. Ray collaborated with other departments to revise hospital policy extending emergency physician orders to sixteen hours, ensuring continuous treatment and pain control for patients while allowing admitting physicians to wait until morning to assess them.

Ray also spoke up when he saw other groups letting their patient care standards slip. The emergency physicians regularly called the gastroenterology service to perform emergency procedures such as removing foreign bodies and identifying sources of internal bleeding. During regular business hours, those patients would go from the emergency room to the gastroenterology suite where they would recover from anesthesia before being discharged. But at night and on the weekends, the patients would return to the emergency room to recover. That overtaxed the emergency room staff, who were stretched too thin to give those patients the attention they deserved. Not wanting his department to be complicit in providing substandard care, Ray collaborated with them on a process for their patients to recover with postsurgical patients or in the intensive care unit rather than the emergency department, relieving them from the additional burden while ensuring the same high standard of care for all post-anesthesia patients.

Two years into his tenure, Ray was still fighting to update the hospital's Code Blue policy. A Code Blue is called for a patient in a life-or-death situation, when seconds count and only skilled assessment and treatment will save their life. Overland Park's Code Blue policy, written in 1993, assigned an emergency physician to the Code Blue team, which responded to crises anywhere in the hospital, both in the emergency rooms and inpatient units. The policy had never been updated to reflect evolving regulations and credentialing requirements.

From the time Ray became medical director in 2012, EmCare never fully staffed the emergency room. If hospital policy stated the emergency physician was responsible for codes, there should have been two emergency physicians on duty at all times. That way, if one was called to attend an inpatient emergency, as they often were, the other would still be present in the emergency room to evaluate patients immediately.

Ray learned in the military that he could use policies, regulations, and legislation as leverage to hold his superiors to their obligations. To protect his physicians from needing to be in multiple places at once, he first warned administrators that Overland Park could lose its classification as a Level II trauma center. That hard-won designation from the American College of Surgeons meant the facility had the expertise to initiate definitive care for all injured patients, but it required that an emergency physician be physically present whenever a traumatically injured patient was in the department. When the American

College of Surgeons made a verification visit to Overland Park in 2014, they flagged the Code Blue policy as a problem but issued no immediate consequences, so EmCare leadership continued to dismiss Ray's concerns, arguing they had until the next visit, which wasn't until 2017, to change staffing. Ray told his administrators the College of Surgeons would look at records from the three intervening years and view the failure to address known deficiencies unfavorably, likely rescinding their Level II status, but EmCare leadership was unfazed.

Ray knew EmCare was courting disaster, both for patients and for the hospital, so he next tried to use financial priorities to convince hospital leaders. The reputation of his emergency room had gotten out in the community and many family doctors steered their sickest patients, who were most likely to need admission, to Overland Park because they knew the care was so good. Losing Level II status would be a blow to the hospital's reputation, and those doctors might send their patients elsewhere. It would also divert ambulances to other facilities and reduce patient volume in the emergency department, which would in turn decrease inpatient bed occupancy because the emergency room was responsible for nearly 85 percent of hospital admissions. But even explaining the potentially catastrophic financial consequences of losing Level II status got Ray nowhere with administrators.

Not long after the verification visit from American College of Surgeons, the hospital expanded the number of emergency and inpatient beds, which eventually totaled 377 — 343 inpatient, 24 adult emergency room, and 10 pediatric emergency room. By 2016, there should have been three emergency physicians on each shift, but EmCare held staffing steady, in keeping with their policy of minimizing overhead, because shareholders were impatient with lackluster returns. Though it hadn't happened yet, Ray knew it was only a matter of time before one of his colleagues faced a nightmare situation — two, or even three, patients in distress, in different locations, and only being able to save one of them — unless he could convince administrators to staff appropriately.

Ray embarked on a methodical campaign to change the Code Blue policy, raising his concerns at every meeting, on every phone call, and in every email he could. He asked for change in terms no one could argue against — patient safety. In one of our conversations, he proudly recounted what one administrator told a colleague about him: "Ray's a bulldog. When he gets something in his teeth, like patient safety, he doesn't let it go."

But all his efforts, and his courage in standing up to a gargantuan bureaucracy, hadn't kept a patient from dying.

EmCare was founded in 1972 at Baylor University Medical Center in Dallas, Texas, by Dr. Leonard Riggs, a former flight surgeon for the navy in Vietnam and a former president of the American College of Emergency Physicians,[6] to help hospitals outsource the time-consuming and largely thankless work of hiring and scheduling a full roster of emergency room physicians. Most were glad for someone else to take on the headache, as evidenced by the explosive growth of EmCare in its first twenty years.

By 1994, when EmCare went public, it had contracts with sixty-one emergency departments in fifteen states.[7] Three years later, Laidlaw, a Canadian company that built school buses and ambulances, acquired EmCare for $336 million, and at the same time acquired American Medical Response, or AMR, an ambulance service company, for $1.25 billion.[8] With Americans growing older and sicker every day, healthcare looked like a recession-proof investment.

State regulators have been clear for decades, though, that money and medical decisions make poor bedfellows. Thirty-three states have laws, some dating back to the nineteenth century, requiring healthcare to be provided by entities owned by licensed clinicians and prohibiting corporations from influencing medical decision making.[9] Hospitals do not engage in medical decision making and therefore can be owned by non-physicians. But for physicians at those hospitals to legally provide healthcare, they need to be officially employed by a separate entity contracted with the hospital to provide physician services. At Dartmouth, where I did my residency, that entity was the Hitchcock Clinic; at Kaiser it is the Permanente Group; at Brigham it is the Brigham and Women's Physicians Organization. Such legal arrangements are the reason patients typically receive separate bills for hospital services and physician services.

EmCare, like other staffing companies, subverted those legal constraints, most commonly by creating subsidiaries with figurehead physician owners. The doctor who "owned" the subsidiary that hired Ray in Kansas, for example, owned a constantly fluctuating number of subsidiaries, hovering around three hundred at any given time across twenty states. In this role, he earned a fixed salary; any profits from the subsidiaries flowed straight through to EmCare.

Laidlaw expanded EmCare from an emergency room staffing company to one that also provided hospitalists and primary care physicians, as well as management services for small hospitals.[10] By 1998, Laidlaw had become one of the leading providers of ambulance and emergency department management services in the United States, but it was losing money on the endeavor. The company had tried to increase profits by scaling back unprofitable contracts and reducing staff, to no avail. Now the subsidiary was dragging down the whole conglomeration.[11]

In 1999, Laidlaw decided to divest from healthcare, to focus on its core business,[12] announcing plans to sell AMR and EmCare and writing off anticipated losses. After two years, the company had yet to find a buyer, so in 2001, Laidlaw filed for bankruptcy.[13] In 2003, with $1.2 billion in financing from Citigroup and Credit Suisse, Laidlaw transferred operations from Canada to the United States and reorganized in Delaware.[14] Finally in 2005, just four years after filing for bankruptcy, Laidlaw sold the AMR and EmCare to a private equity firm, Onex Partners, for $828 million, a substantial loss tempered by the write-off in 1999.[15]

Private equity firms like Onex Partners pool money from diverse sources — such as university endowments, insurance companies, pension plans, or very wealthy individuals — and invest it in under-performing companies, with the express intent of maximizing the return on that investment for shareholders, usually in the range of 20 to 30 percent, within three to five years. When private equity firms invest in any company, they typically seek a voice in the decisions the company makes, whether through seats on the board or by installing a handpicked management team, and they employ a variety of tactics to reduce overhead and increase revenue in order to turn a quick profit on their investments.

Management teams, almost always headed by business experts with MBAs, are taught to scour the balance sheet for overlooked inefficiencies, starting with the largest cost center. In most healthcare organizations, human resources is the largest expense, so when Onex invested in EmCare, new managers looked to cut personnel, hours, or wages, and to hire less experienced, less extensively trained staff that cost one-third to one-half as much. A 2022 study by the National Bureau of Economic Research found that having an MBA in charge of a company, rather than a non-MBA, led to a 6 percent drop in wages over five years, and a reduction in the amount of corporate revenue dedicated to wages of 5 percent.[16]

To increase revenue, private equity employs several strategies, including some that are ethically and legally questionable in a medical setting. Onex Partners owned more than 80 percent of voting shares in EmCare when the staffing company got in trouble for pressuring doctors in HMA hospitals to document patients as sicker than they were to justify a higher billing code and better reimbursement, a practice known as upcoding.[17] Another tactic, "surprise billing," has garnered a great deal of attention in recent years for inflicting harrowing financial toxicity on patients. When patients visit an emergency room at a hospital that is in-network with their insurance company, they have no reason to suspect that the emergency room physicians are out-of-network and therefore not covered by their insurance. But if the staffing company elects not to contract with local insurers, they can then surprise patients with direct bills for as much as they want to charge. Patients, who usually didn't even know they were getting out-of-network care or had no choice, because of emergency response constraints that require transport to the nearest facility, have no recourse when presented with such a bill.[18]

Companies also insert language into contracts to maximize the revenue they can extract from employees. Non-solicitation clauses, like the one that kept Matt Ramsey from telling me where he was moving, are designed to make it hard for physicians to leave staffing companies to work for competitors. Non-compete clauses, which Tristán Associates dealt with in chapter 11, keep physicians from working within a certain radius for a specified length of time, typically one to two years. Such clauses, while not always enforceable, may be expensive to fight, and are harmful both to clinicians, who face uprooting their families to find eligible opportunities, and to patients, who may subsequently struggle to access care.

In 2011, Onex sold EmCare, and AMR, known together as Emergency Medical Services Corporation, to another private equity company, Clayton, Dubilier & Rice, in a $3.2 billion deal.[19] With this final sale, after selling shares piecemeal over several years and settling its debts, Onex realized $1.65 billion in profits, nearly eight times its original investment of $214 million.[20] At Clayton, Dubilier & Rice, EmCare became part of a multibillion-dollar corporation whose advisers included moguls from General Electric, Boeing, Disney, Emerson Electric, The Gap, IBM, PepsiCo, Procter & Gamble, and Unilever. EmCare was no longer in the hands of physicians or anyone else with patient care as a priority. It was a "diversification asset" in a huge corporate portfolio, expected to carry its weight alongside every other industry.

A month after the sale, and shortly before Ray joined EmCare, EmCare entered into the previously mentioned joint venture with HCA, the country's largest hospital corporation, to staff its emergency rooms.[21] Because EmCare had been staffing emergency rooms at a number of HCA hospitals for some time, analysts weren't immediately clear on why the two corporations would enter into this new relationship rather than continue their previous contracting arrangement. Some speculated it was to hide kickbacks, especially as allegations of such illegal behavior were beginning to swirl around EmCare's relationships with other hospital corporations, like HMA from chapter 2.[22] Another theory was inspired by the fact that EmCare was precariously burdened with debt. A joint venture structure would have allowed EmCare to access additional resources from a company with substantial tangible assets against which to borrow, while HCA in turn could exert outsized control over its primary staffing contractor.

Either way, EmCare was powerfully motivated to keep HCA's $1.5 billion of business. That meant HCA had leverage to coerce physicians under EmCare's direction and control to behave in HCA's interests — increasing admissions, ordering more tests, documenting patients as sicker than they were, or tolerating understaffing.[23] For Ray to speak up, he would have to take on not just his local or regional leadership, but the whole massive machine of HCA and EmCare together.

When the patient died at Overland Park, Ray escalated his concerns up his leadership chain quickly, sending an email on July 30 to Dr. Patrick McHugh, an EmCare executive vice president responsible for all hospital contracts in the Greater Kansas City region, expressing concern on behalf of all the emergency physicians. Within days his team was granted a meeting with Dr. McHugh, but no changes resulted. A few weeks later, Dr. McHugh sent an email to the emergency physicians at Overland Park explaining EmCare's position: "HCA is a for-profit company traded on the New York Stock Exchange. Many of their staffing decisions are financially motivated. EmCare is no different. Profits are in everyone's best interest."[24]

In September, Ray composed a letter "communicating that the entire group of physicians who provide emergency services at Overland

Park were very concerned about the Code Blue policy affecting their ability to provide safe, timely care to the emergency room patients because they were required to be in potentially three places at once." The letter also "expressed the growing anxiety that emergency room physicians were experiencing as a result of the policy."[25] All twenty-two of the emergency physicians who worked for him reviewed and signed the letter. On September 30, 2017, he sent the letter to Dr. McHugh, hopeful that McHugh might use it to fight for change with his leadership, but McHugh did not reply. Weeks later, when their paths crossed, Ray asked if he'd received the letter, to which McHugh responded, "Why would you ever put that in writing?"

A few months after their encounter in the hallway, on Tuesday, January 17, 2017, Dr. McHugh invited Ray to dinner. Ray thought the dinner might be about the negotiations he was leading for the first pay raise in six years for his physicians and physician assistants, but he wasn't sure. Having never trusted McHugh and, feeling like his back was against the wall, Ray recorded the meeting, heedless of whether it was legal under Kansas law to do so without the other party's consent. Fortunately for Ray, it was.

During the meal, McHugh dismissed him from his duties at Overland Park. Ray was, in his words, "more oppositional than supportive" of EmCare policies and was causing trouble because he "kept fighting against things." "You cash the check every month to be a corporate representative," McHugh admonished him, "and there is a responsibility . . . to support the corporation's objectives."[26] Before he left, McHugh mentioned that EmCare might have other work for him as a medical director at a hospital ninety minutes away in Clinton, Missouri.

When he got home, Ray asked his wife to help him draft a letter to the director of human resources to complain about his removal. "I fear that [Dr. McHugh's] actions are in retaliation for my constant concerns voiced respectfully about patient safety issues," he wrote. "That was part of my job as director. There does not appear to be any other grounds for these actions."[27] Though her read receipt indicated she'd opened it, the human resources director never replied to the message. When Ray's lawyers later obtained her emails in preparation for the trial, he learned that within three minutes of receiving the email she forwarded it to McHugh. The next morning, McHugh rescinded the offer of a position in Clinton and told Ray he would not be allowed to work anywhere in the Mid America Division, which included all the EmCare contracted hospitals within commuting distance. The day after he got fired, Ray retained a lawyer to help him make his case against EmCare.

Watching Ray get fired for speaking up had a chilling effect on the Overland Park emergency department. For several months, his former colleagues, many of whom were younger physicians with student loan debt, kept their heads down, "petrified" of retaliation if they spoke up again about patient safety concerns. Determined to show his colleagues, both at Overland Park and in other emergency departments across the country, that their efforts to protect patients were not in vain, on April 27, 2017, Ray filed a lawsuit accusing EmCare subsidiaries that employed him, KS-I and MO-I Medical Services, of wrongful discharge in violation of public policy, alleging "the reason his employment was terminated as Medical Director and emergency room physician was because of his complaints of dangerous and illegal understaffing of the Overland Park emergency department."[28] In suing for millions in damages, Ray stood to make an enormous sum if he won, but as he told me, "The money was secondary." "I had to stand up and do the right thing, because I have to believe the good guy — and patients — will win out in the end."

Ray's approach to his trial was to hire the best lawyers he could, give them all the information he had, and let them do their work. He recalled one of his lawyers telling him at the start, "Let us worry about this. You go take care of your family." Ray took that advice to heart. "The more I put the whole business on the back burner, the better off I was," he told me in reflection.

The trial began in September 2018. After eight days in court, the jury deliberated for two hours and found in favor of Ray, awarding him $2,817,045 in economic damages, $6 million in non-economic damages for pain and suffering, and $20 million in punitive damages. But the case wasn't settled just yet. A Kansas court reduced his award by misapplying a law that capped judgments, and Ray's lawyers encouraged him to appeal. In March 2021, after more than three years of litigation, a judge restored $26 million of his original $29 million award.

While he was battling EmCare in court, Ray took a job with a group of emergency physicians who formerly worked for EmCare but whose contract McHugh had recently ended. Under Ray's leadership, the physicians formed their own private, democratically organized group and negotiated a contract with the same hospital EmCare had stopped staffing. For two years, the group had no turnover and similar performance metrics to the Overland Park group. After the hospital abruptly chose to hire another contract group, Ray worked at temporary positions for the remainder of his trial. From afar, he watched with pride as all his Overland Park colleagues eventually found the courage to leave. The new director lasted just twelve months; the eighteen other emergency physicians who had worked with Ray, some of whom had been at Overland Park for more than a decade, either left the facility to work at another EmCare location or left the corporation entirely.

Because of the judgment, Ray will be financially secure for the rest of his life. But instead of retiring from medicine, he decided to set up an infusion clinic for the treatment of depression. For the first time in his career, he's practicing medicine as he believes it should be done — hourlong appointments, holistic conversations, with no computers or clocks standing in the way of human connection. After being open for a year, many patients have already told him he's changed their lives, and he knows the experience with them has changed his. Running his own clinic confirms Ray's hunch that allowing doctors, rather than corporations, to control how they care for patients is better for everyone. He's grateful for the opportunity to heal his community and to recover from his own brush with moral injury.

From 2000 to 2018, private equity investment in healthcare increased from $5 billion to $100 billion. Today private-equity-owned staffing companies like EmCare, renamed Envision in 2013, TeamHealth (Blackstone Group), SCP Health (Onex Corporation, which sold EmCare in 2011), and US Acute Care Services (Welsh, Carson, Anderson, and Stowe) control about 40 percent of emergency room staffing in the country. Nearly half of doctors responsible for treating some of the most vulnerable patients in society are employed by corporations whose explicit goal is to maximize shareholder profit. Because these companies have become so prevalent, in some regions they are the only option for employment as an emergency physician. As a result, many physicians despair at finding somewhere they can practice medicine in alignment with their values.

The story of Ray Brovont shows there is another way. By choosing to work for EmCare, excelling in his role as medical director, and systematically holding his employer to account for putting profits before patients, Ray laid the groundwork for a public fight that he was prepared to win. He stood up for his patients and his fellow clinicians, claiming victory for them and for the profession of medicine.

A Transformational Leader

In December 2020, after two brutal surges of the coronavirus without vaccines, many healthcare workers cried tears of relief when they
got their vaccinations. They could finally protect themselves and their
families from infection, and they expected widespread immunization
would mean fewer critically ill patients overwhelming their hospitals.

When large segments of society, even some healthcare workers,
bought into baseless conspiratorial rhetoric and opted out of vaccination once they were eligible, clinicians who had gotten the jab,
including many doctors, were angry. They felt betrayed and taken for
granted by the very people they had risked their lives to protect, and
they braced themselves for the inevitable next surge if vaccine uptake
didn't increase.

Physicians at hospitals like the University of Florida Health
Jacksonville that serve primarily low-income populations were especially worried about how their patients would weather another surge.
With less access to care, disproportionate rates of chronic illnesses,
and low vaccination rates, their patients were at high risk of becoming
severely ill if they caught the virus.

Dr. Mark McIntosh, the medical director for employee wellness
at UF Health Jacksonville, knew from reading our work that the
distress he was witnessing in his workforce was a kind of moral injury.
He thought it might help his team if they had better language to
describe their experience, so in April 2021, he invited me to speak
to the university's College of Medicine. About forty participants
attended the virtual talk introducing them to the concept. "I agree

that systemic changes need to be made to address moral injury," one participant wrote on their feedback form to the organizers, "but we as physicians are not empowered to make them right now. This topic should be presented to our administrative leadership." Mark agreed, so he passed information about our work to Dr. Leon Haley Jr., who served as both dean of the College of Medicine and CEO of UF Health Jacksonville.

The following month, Dr. Haley asked Mark to find out if I could facilitate a workshop at their executive retreat in June. Despite the short notice, I immediately agreed, eager to do something tangible to help alleviate the distress I saw building to alarming levels in too many hospitals.

For my first virtual meeting with Leon and his team a few weeks before the retreat, I prepared the kind of crisp briefing I usually delivered to executives who are overloaded with information and short on time. During introductions, Leon was energetic and gregarious, putting everyone at ease with a bit of levity. But when we started talking about his staff, he became quiet and pensive. He chose his words carefully and his brow creased ever so slightly. It's a look I've seen on physicians' faces when their patients aren't doing well; he was worried.

Leon told me that despite dedicating significant resources to addressing burnout — such as opening the Center for Healthy Minds and Practice to provide free on-campus behavioral health resources in 2019 — he knew his clinicians were still suffering, and not just because of the pandemic. When I explained what I meant by moral injury, and how it differed from burnout, Leon grasped the concept immediately, having worked for years as an emergency room physician. We talked well past the end of our scheduled time about the sources of distress at UF Health Jacksonville — previous leaders had been indecisive and slow to act, and for too long, clinicians felt no one had been looking out for them — and what he and his administrative staff could do to help. A few days later, when I had questions about background material he had sent, he personally took my call.

For the in-person retreat in Jacksonville in mid-June, Leon brought together about twenty people, including the chair of each department, his chief operating officer, who was also a doctor, and a few administrators who worked closely with the physicians. During the sessions, Leon sat in the back of the room, listening carefully but letting the doctors have the floor. At one point, I asked the physicians whether they'd prefer if he stepped out of the room for a bit. Their response was unanimous — he should stay. His physicians saw him as one of them and trusted him enough to be frank.

At the end of the meeting, Leon offered to drive me the ten minutes to my hotel. After opening the passenger door for me, he settled into the driver's seat, running a clearly practiced, methodical internal checklist before driving off — sunglasses just so, visor in place, scan each mirror — while cheerfully recounting his boyhood in Pittsburgh, Pennsylvania. By the end of that short trip, I sensed I had found the final story I needed for the book, about an executive at a larger health system who led in partnership with the physicians he served.

After I returned home, we exchanged a few emails, promising to regroup later in the summer to consider next steps after we both had a bit of time to reflect on how the group responded to the engagement. Over the following weeks, I thought often of Leon and his staff as North Florida faced its third, and worst, surge of the pandemic, which threatened to overwhelm the region's hospitals.

Then on Monday, July 26, I received an email from Mark telling me that Dean Haley had died over the weekend. Two days before, Leon was piloting a Jet Ski in Palm Beach, Florida, when he lost control and crashed into a rock jetty. Witnesses and the responding Coast Guard crew tried to resuscitate him on the way to St. Mary's Hospital in West Palm Beach, but his injuries were grave, and he died shortly after his arrival at the hospital. Such an unexpected death would have been tragic at any time, but losing their champion during a massive coronavirus surge, when they needed him most, left his staff reeling.

I had already been planning to include Leon's story in this book, but I didn't get the chance to interview him in depth before he died, so I spoke with his loved ones, colleagues, and employees and reviewed hours of online videos of him and of memorial services held in his honor. His colleagues and staff remembered him as attentive, reflective, generous, and steady, with a huge smile ready at the slightest provocation. He earned their respect because he showed up for them, and even more important, he fought for them.

Leon Leroy Haley Jr. grew up in the Point Breeze neighborhood of Pittsburgh in the 1960s. Established in the late nineteenth century by magnates like Henry Heinz, George Westinghouse, and Andrew Carnegie, during Leon's childhood Point Breeze still featured wide streets and many of the original mansions, though some had been torn down to make way for higher-density housing. His mother, Elizabeth Ann, stayed home while Leon, his brother, and his sister were young, then earned her education degree and began teaching in public schools. After starting his career as a probation officer for Alleghany County, his father, Leon Sr., taught public policy at a series of historically Black colleges.

When Leon was in high school, his father became president and CEO of the Urban League of Pittsburgh, the largest social services organization serving the Black community in southwestern Pennsylvania, before returning to academia to earn tenure at the University of Pittsburgh. The Haleys spent a lot of time around the dinner table and in the AME Zion church congregation every Sunday talking with their children about how their privilege came with the responsibility to help others. As Leon Sr. put it when we spoke, they taught their children to serve "the least, the lost, and the left behind."

His parents enrolled Leon and his brother at Shady Side Academy, a prestigious private school just five minutes from their home, with a reputation for encouraging their students to get involved in their community. Leon Sr. often told his children, in preparing them to become activists: "It doesn't matter how good your ideas are, if you can't communicate them effectively." At Shady Side, where he played varsity football, Leon became a strong writer and public speaker. His goal was to work in broadcasting until he tried a trick basketball dunk from a trampoline and tore the cartilage in his knee. Fascinated by his encounters with the surgeon who repaired his knee and his experience as a patient in the hospital, he decided to become an orthopedic surgeon instead.

From Shady Side, Leon went to Brown University, where he majored in biology. Providence was too far from Pittsburgh for a weekend trip, so during college he started what became a lifelong habit of calling home every Sunday to stay connected with his family and where he came from. For medical school, he chose the University of Pittsburgh to minimize his debt — as a public school, the tuition was relatively low, and he could live with his parents, who were thrilled to have him back.

The summer after his first year of medical school, Leon joined a program to give medical students more clinical experience. For two months he rotated through general surgery, the emergency department, and primary care. As he later recalled to a group of young people in a leadership seminar, "I was in the operating room with a gown on, mask on, gloved . . . and my ADD would kick in and I just couldn't stand there anymore."[1] To his surprise, he found himself drawn not to surgery but to emergency medicine, where the urgent pace was a better match for his personality and where he felt he could make the most impact on the disadvantaged populations his parents encouraged him to serve.

While in medical school, Leon met Carla, a fellow student one year behind him who had studied psychology and run track at Penn State University. She shared his commitment to community and a passion for sports — in particular, Penn State football. They married at the end of Leon's fourth year, just before he moved to Detroit for his three-year emergency medicine residency at Henry Ford Hospital;

Carla joined him there the following year for her four-year, combined internal medicine-pediatrics residency. Though Detroit was once the booming Motor City, by the time he arrived in 1990, rates of unemployment, poverty per capita, infant mortality, homicide, and homelessness were among the highest in the country, and the city had become known as Murder City, USA.[2]

Leon chose Henry Ford in part because it is a "safety-net" hospital, a designation the Institute of Medicine assigns to facilities that provide a significant level of healthcare to uninsured patients or those with Medicaid; because the federal government deems their services "essential," most safety-net hospitals receive some public funding.[3] At Henry Ford, Leon thought, he would see the worst of everything emergency medicine could throw at him, while serving those most in need of care.

Leon's idealism faded quickly once he started residency. While he felt his work in the emergency room had meaning and purpose, by his second year he already realized "how broken healthcare was." But rather than despairing, he vowed to do something about it.[4] When Leon finished residency in 1993 and took a position as an attending emergency physician at Henry Ford, Carla still had two years of training left. Because she would be at the hospital day and night anyway, Leon decided to spend his nights and one weekend each month in Ann Arbor, a forty-five-minute drive west of Detroit, studying public health, hospital operations, and business administration to earn a master of health services administration degree from the University of Michigan. When Carla finished her residency in 1995, she took a job in Detroit, and in early January 1996, the first of their three children was born.

In 1997, Leon, restless for more responsibility, made a cold call to Dr. Art Kellermann, the founding chairman of emergency medicine at Emory University in Atlanta, about a possible job at Grady Hospital, a safety-net hospital affiliated with the university. Grady served a similar patient population to Henry Ford, but it was much larger and offered more leadership opportunities. Leon also thought Kellermann, who was well known in the field of public health — his research focused on gun safety and the role of emergency departments in care for the poor — might be an ideal mentor. In that first conversation, Art invited Leon to apply for the position of chief of emergency medicine. After several rounds of application reviews and in-person interviews during which Leon's poise and preparation shone, Dr. Kellermann offered him the job. Leon, after persuading Carla to leave Detroit, accepted.

About a year after he started at Grady, Leon Sr. visited Atlanta, and Leon showed him the challenges he faced in an urban emergency room. "If you have money, whether you're Black or white, you just don't go to Grady," he told his father as they walked through a hallway overflowing with patient beds. "This place serves the poorest of the poor." Leon shook his head, remarking, "Our society is so violent, there's just not enough room for everyone who's harmed." He was determined to make more room so Grady physicians could treat those patients with the dignity he thought they deserved.

But budgets are always tight at public hospitals, so Leon couldn't just expand the emergency room, as the HCA-owned, for-profit Overland Park Regional Medical Center did in chapter 12. Before coming up with a strategy, Leon knew he needed to hear from the patients they served, so he led Grady's participation in a multi-hospital study analyzing the various reasons patients used the emergency room. Emergency rooms have a high concentration of sophisticated, lifesaving equipment and experts ready to deploy at a moment's notice, which makes them expensive to run. Health systems had long assumed that patients turned to emergency rooms only as a last resort, but the researchers found that about one-third of emergency visits were not emergencies at all. Rather, patients turned to the emergency room because they had no other options for care.[5] Armed with this data, Leon developed a low-cost plan to relieve the financial strain on the emergency department and free up space.

The first part of his plan was to redouble efforts to triage minor problems like an earache, small cut, or sprained ankle to the urgent care center adjacent to the emergency room. By retraining staff about criteria for urgent care visits and having the charge nurse audit charts several times each shift to make sure patients were being seen in the appropriate place, he reduced emergency department volume by roughly one-third. Next, he relocated the urgent care patient charts from the main emergency room information desk to the urgent care area, so clinicians could easily see how many patients were waiting and quickly move through the simplest cases, which reduced the urgent care's waiting time from 214 to 94 minutes and increased its productivity by one-third, from an average of fifty-one patients seen each day to sixty-seven.[6]

Sometimes patients arrive at the emergency room with symptoms that do not qualify for hospital admission but are nonetheless worrisome. Sending these patients straight home often led them to return within days for the same problem, a process the Institute of Medicine called avoidable readmissions. But keeping people in the emergency room for observation, known as boarding, ties up beds and pulls nursing resources from patients in crisis.[7] Other times emergency departments board patients simply because they face obstacles to discharging them — the patients are unhoused, are unable to pick up their medications, or lack access to home health services. Leon tackled both boarding and readmissions by setting up a dedicated team, the Care Management Unit, that combined an observation stay unit with intensive case management support, reducing the emergency department readmission rate by nearly 30 percent.[8]

These changes were not only good for patients and for clinicians, but they also helped the hospital's bottom line. Between the slight increase in revenue from the urgent care center and the Care Management Unit, plus the reduced costs of caring for patients in lower acuity settings, Grady realized a net benefit of $190 million.

While at Grady, Leon had ample opportunity to learn from the examples of other leaders, both good and bad, who tried various tactics to get the deeply indebted hospital back on solid financial ground. After five CEOs in three years, Grady's board of directors brought in Mike Young, the same leader who later ran Pinnacle Health during its contract with Tristán Associates from chapter 11. Young, who had no clinical background, was brought in for his financial savvy, and he delivered, turning an $80 million annual loss into a $25 million gain by his second year.

To produce such a quick turnaround, Young slashed three hundred jobs in his first year, closed three of the nine neighborhood clinics residents relied on for their preventive care, and shuttered Grady's dialysis clinic, all without seeking input from the community. He also tightened rules about income, identification, and residence verification required to qualify for discounted care, so patients without pay stubs, who were unemployed or paid in cash, were ineligible. While limiting access to discounted care saved the hospital money, at least in the short term, it meant more patients were forced to use the emergency room as their only primary care option, and had more preventable health crises, both of which distressed the physicians who cared for them.

In Young, Leon witnessed what happened to a powerful man who was heedless of his privilege. At a breakfast meeting in October 2010, Young told Atlanta business leaders that because he'd saved taxpayers so much money, the poor, largely Black, Fulton County residents "should want to shine my shoes." That racially insensitive comment was the beginning of the end for Young at Grady, though it didn't deter Pinnacle Health from bringing him to Pennsylvania in March 2011.[9]

When Young left, the Grady board looked for "a healer,"[10] hiring John Haupert as the new CEO. He had been the chief operating officer at Parkland Memorial, a public hospital of comparable size in Dallas, Texas. While Haupert, like Young, lacked clinical experience, he knew his job was to serve clinicians. A self-described consensus builder, Haupert spent months listening to the staff and the community before making changes, and Leon was impressed by how he took their concerns seriously.[11]

Whereas Young focused on cutting costs, even if doing so undermined the organization's mission to serve disadvantaged populations as a safety-net hospital, Haupert focused on inclusive growth and building a health system clinicians could be proud to be part of. In his first five years, he created or expanded programs in cardiac care, urology, orthopedic surgery, stroke, trauma, and burns, which attracted more privately insured patients, from 12 to 20 percent. He began a comprehensive program to help uninsured patients sign up for Medicaid, decreasing the proportion of uninsured patients at Grady from 42 percent to 27 percent. Those measures helped Grady retain previously uninsured or underinsured patients, who historically sought care at "better" hospitals once they qualified for Medicare, which every local hospital accepted. According to Mike King, a longtime Atlanta journalist and author of the book *A Spirit of Charity: Restoring the Bond Between America and Its Public Hospitals*, Haupert did "a remarkable job of not just holding [Grady] together, but renewing and stabilizing its essential role in the community and state."[12]

Haupert also made Grady a better place to visit and to work by updating and expanding hospital infrastructure, funded by an eight-year, $350 million fundraising campaign, started by Mike Young.[13] Ensuring that clinicians have the tools and the resources they need to do their jobs well is central to reducing the potential for moral injury. Knowing leadership is fighting for those resources does the same. Although I never asked Leon about his mentors, during a leadership talk he gave his second year in Jacksonville, he acknowledged John Haupert was a powerful influence.[14]

While at Grady, Leon and Carla welcomed two more children. Despite his demanding career, Leon made his children a priority. As he did with his colleagues and as he learned from his mentors, he challenged his children to find what they were passionate about, surround themselves with smart people and listen to them, and take calculated risks to grow. Although all three were gifted athletes like their parents, Leon and Carla also taught them that sports were a means to a university degree that would allow them to give back to the world.

In July 2013, Grady entered a closer contractual relationship with the Emory University School of Medicine, and Leon was promoted to two new roles: executive associate dean of the School of Medicine and deputy senior vice president of medical affairs at Grady. Leon would be the chief liaison between Emory and Grady, providing executive leadership, strategic vision, and direction for Emory's clinical, research, and teaching activities at Grady Hospital. After more than a decade at Grady, Leon was finally moving into the leadership role he'd envisioned on those weekend trips from Detroit to Ann Arbor.

Three years into his tenure at Emory, Leon was still learning his roles and busy cheering on his three children at their games — at this point, his oldest, who would go on to play in the NFL, was playing college football at Penn State — when his name came up as a potential candidate for the newly vacant position as dean of the School of Medicine at the University of Florida in Jacksonville.

David Vukich, the chief medical officer at UF Health Jacksonville and the chair of the search committee, had never heard of Leon, but on the advice of a colleague who had followed Leon's career, David cold-called him to gauge his interest. The UF Health Jacksonville system was huge: It included two of the state's nine academic medical centers, supported nearly twenty thousand jobs, and generated $2.874 billion in revenue.[15] Running it would be a formidable challenge and would require someone with an uncommon set of attributes.

The city of Jacksonville covers an area of 840 square miles, the largest landmass of any city in the contiguous United States.[16] Nearly one million residents from diverse backgrounds — half white, one-third Black, one-tenth Latino — live in the "River City," so named for the St. John's River that flows north to the Atlantic Ocean, dividing the city geographically and socioeconomically. One in seven people lives in poverty, slightly lower than the average for cities in the United States, and about the same number are uninsured.[17]

With eighteen hospitals inside the city limits, including a satellite of Mayo Clinic, two HCA facilities, a navy hospital, and a Veterans Affairs facility, in addition to UF Health Jacksonville's two academic medical centers, healthcare is big business in Jacksonville. In that mix of hospitals, UF Health Jacksonville was the only safety-net facility, and most years, the system provided around $250 million in charity care, one of largest contributions in the state.[18]

Both low-income and wealthy patients worried they would get lesser care from safety-net hospitals, colloquially known by the misnomer "providers of last resort." Wealthier patients shunned UF Health Jacksonville hospital in favor of "nicer," though not necessarily more expert, private institutions, and took their high-reimbursement insurance coverage with them, which reinforced the distrust low-income patients already felt towards the hospital as their only option for care. Many health systems subsidize uninsured or underinsured care with revenue from better-reimbursing private insurance, and not being able to do so meant UF Health Jacksonville had to find the money elsewhere. The city of Jacksonville paid the health system $26 million annually to care for its citizens living below the poverty line, but that still left a roughly $50 million hole in the institution's revenue. The state legislature often pledged to fill in gaps, but funding was approved at unpredictable intervals, so the health system's finances were perpetually unstable.[19]

From the first time they talked, David sensed that Leon was just what Jacksonville needed. Reflecting on that conversation, he recounted to me, wistfully, "You always felt better after talking to Leon than you did when you started." When Leon met the search committee, he "hit it out of the park." "He was confident but not arrogant, charismatic but genuine. No matter what they asked him about, he had an answer, because he'd seen it all before: issues of racism, community relations, engaging philanthropy, dealing with local and state politics, advocacy."

Shortly after his trip to Gainesville late in the summer, the board made an offer, which Leon accepted. On January 1, 2017, Dr. Haley became Dean Haley of the UF Jacksonville College of Medicine, VP of health affairs, and professor of emergency medicine. A few months later, he would add CEO of UF Health Jacksonville to his responsibilities — the first African American physician to hold those titles, and the first person to combine the roles.

When he became CEO, Leon took on a health system with a large uninsured population, an image problem with the wealthier citizens of Jacksonville, weak connections to other health systems and businesses in the area, minimal philanthropic support, and a demoralized workforce. With challenges so interconnected, to make progress in any one area, Leon would have to tackle them all.

When I spoke with David Vukich, I asked him what Leon was like as a leader. "He wasn't afraid of anything," David recalled. "The hard job? 'Give it to me.' Have to stay up late? 'I'll take it.' Have to work weekends? 'Sign me up.' He never asked more of his colleagues than he asked of himself." Perhaps most critical to his effectiveness, he never lost sight of the fact that his job was to serve clinicians.

When Leon arrived at UF Health Jacksonville in January, the organization was deep into Phase Two of an expansion project designed to better serve the city's growing and aging population. Two years earlier, the health system had opened a new medical office building that also housed an emergency room and an ambulatory surgery center. The second stage of the project was an adjacent ninety-two-bed inpatient tower, including twenty beds for women's services, a twenty-four-bed intensive care unit, and forty-eight general medical inpatient beds, slated to open in May.[20] The previous administration had not made staffing the new tower a priority, which frustrated staff at existing sites, who feared being pressured to work overtime, further straining their capacity to serve their own patients.

After meeting Leon, and learning of his dynamic leadership at

Grady, David had expected him to be his wingman in tense meetings with the current staff about temporarily taking on extra shifts in the new hospital, since there wasn't time to hire enough staff before the opening. But Leon wasn't moved to premature action by David's anxiety. Following the example of John Haupert at Grady, Leon sat quietly and listened, making sure he understood the concerns of all the stakeholders involved. Then he built cohesion with staff, one radically transparent faculty meeting at a time and through countless individual conversations, around the mission of the hospital — "to heal, to comfort, to educate and to discover"[21] — and his broader vision of the organization's direction and goals. When he shared a detailed recruitment plan for the new hospital and asked his physicians for a six-month commitment to fill in gaps in the new facility's schedule, they understood why he was asking and trusted the commitment would be time-limited.

But Leon knew it wasn't enough to tell his staff he valued them. When he became CEO in September 2017, he made it his top strategic priority to secure more resources, so his clinicians would face fewer barriers when caring for patients. Leon recognized community stakeholders as potential sources of support and collaboration, so he invested in relationships with groups such as the Jacksonville Chamber of Commerce, the Jacksonville Civic Council, the American Hospital Association Urban Sustainability Committee, the Florida Hospital Association, the Florida Safety Net Hospital Alliance, and the Jacksonville Electric Authority. He joked, when I saw him, that he hadn't eaten dinner at his own house for weeks because every night when he wasn't traveling, he was at a dinner with one of these stakeholders.

One such partnership was with the nearby military hospital, Naval Hospital Jacksonville, to provide training for navy corpsmen and surgeons. As an urban Level I trauma center, UF Health Jacksonville offered the closest simulation of battlefield conditions possible outside of a conflict zone.[22] During the training program, navy corpsmen spent two weeks at Naval Hospital Jacksonville followed by five weeks at UF Health Jacksonville, rotating through learning modules in wound management, the emergency department, trauma resuscitation, and intensive care.[23] The partnership also allowed navy trauma surgeons to practice at UF Jacksonville's hospitals to maintain certain skills they learned in residency, such as robotic surgery, which Naval Hospital Jacksonville did not perform. Building that bridge endowed UF Health Jacksonville with additional credibility in a region with strong military and veteran presence and expanded opportunities for collaboration in Department of Defense medical research grants.

In 2018, Leon persuaded Jacksonville's mayor, Lenny Curry, to allocate additional city funds, $15 million in 2019, and another $120 million over the subsequent five years, to upgrade and improve the city-owned hospital's fire suppression system, generators, air-conditioning, roofs, and operating rooms, some of which were long overdue for repairs.[24] The updates not only made the hospital a more pleasant place to work but also meant his staff no longer had to worry whether they would have reliable backup power for ventilators, IV pumps, and operating room lights during the hurricanes that routinely hit the region.

Securing more resources was only one part of moving UF Health Jacksonville toward financial stability. Leon worked tirelessly to attract more privately insured patients by promoting UF Health Jacksonville as being on the cutting edge of innovation and establishing high-visibility, high-quality care teams for common conditions, very much like John Haupert had done at Grady.

In tackling each challenge, Leon recognized that his workforce was his most valuable asset. From regular surveys, he knew many of his staff felt stressed and overwhelmed by the challenges of working with such a disadvantaged population in a resource-constrained environment. Shortly after becoming CEO, he charged Mark McIntosh, his medical director for employee wellness, with developing a strategic plan for addressing burnout and improving well-being and resilience. Mark chose a group of physicians to form a task force, and Leon approved protected time off from their clinical duties to participate. The task force envisioned a Center for Healthy Minds and Practice with extended hours to accommodate clinician shifts, which would offer free on-campus behavioral health resources, among other forms of support. The proposed cost was significant — nearly half a million dollars — but Leon approved it immediately. The center opened in the spring of 2019 and has supported the UF Health Jacksonville community through the pandemic, Leon's death, and other tragedies in the healthcare community.

In my years of work on moral injury, I have yet to hear of another executive greenlighting so much money, on the spot, for clinician well-being, let alone insisting that those clinicians be the ones who decide how to spend it. As Mark said in an email to me, "He was like no leader I had ever experienced. He was willing to listen and take risks."

When the pandemic hit in early 2020, Leon braced himself to lead the organization through the crisis. His first step was to double down on his existing strategy of transparent, consistent communication. Whereas previously he recorded short videos for his staff every two weeks with updates on progress toward strategic goals and other issues, during virus surges he shot a video every day so that, in his words, "at least at the end of the day, they would know, here's how we're doing, here's the expertise, here's what's happening, here's 'the struggle.'"

In December 2020, UF Health Jacksonville was chosen as one of the first five hospitals to receive the Pfizer vaccine in the state of Florida. The goal was to vaccinate as many front-line workers as possible, but Leon knew that would not be easy. When he surveyed his staff, he learned that only 40 percent of his team were willing to take the vaccine. After an extensive education campaign, he still had staff reaching out to him with concerns and asking if he was going to take the vaccine. "I made an executive decision," he told the *New England Journal of Medicine Catalyst Innovations in Healthcare Delivery*, "to say 'All right, I will take it, and go first and show my team that I'm comfortable taking the vaccine. I understand the commitment that's behind it. I understand the research behind it.'" He also wanted to inspire confidence in the vaccine among the Black community in Florida. The strategy worked: Immediately after his vaccination was televised, vaccination signups at the hospital doubled.

When I attended the retreat that June weekend, I asked Leon during a break how often he visited the emergency room or walked the floors of the hospital. It's a question I regularly pose to executives, to gauge their exposure to the realities of the front line. Often the response is once or twice a month. Occasionally, executives confess to being in clinical spaces as infrequently as once a year. Leon told me he parked his car in the parking lot across from the emergency room every morning, then walked through the department on the way to his office as a way of taking the pulse of his organization. If the emergency department was overflowing, it was an early warning sign that there was trouble — such as a crisis in the community or understaffing — that he needed to confront before conditions got out of hand. Leon also walked through each inpatient unit almost every week, taking a minute to talk with anyone he encountered, whether clinician, environmental services, or dietary support, about their day and their challenges.

One of the topics that came up in conversations with clinicians in almost every department was money. Many of the clinicians at UF Health Jacksonville had come to equate their salaries, which were lower than those of clinicians in private systems, with their value. At the retreat, Leon asked me if I had any thoughts on how he could help his workforce see the benefits of their work. As a lifelong employee of safety-net institutions himself, he genuinely believed the satisfaction of serving those in need was more than enough to offset the salary difference, and he wanted his employees to feel the same. As he said about his leadership style to the *Jacksonville Business Journal* when they awarded him their Ultimate CEO and Legacy Award in 2019, "I want people to see the big picture and their role in helping the organization achieve a greater good, and not just see it through their eyes."[25] In addition to sharing why he chose a career in safety-net hospitals, I suggested he explain the financial benefits of being a public employee, such as ample pensions, that his staff might have overlooked.

At the end of retreat, we started drafting a plan to address moral injury at UF Health Jacksonville: continuing his effort to shift the organizational culture by listening to front-line workers and communicating transparently, building on the strengths of the organization, and most of all teaching department chairs how to be advocates so they could lead their teams by example. If Leon were still alive, I am confident he would have carried it out.

Like Priya Mammen's mentor Dr. Vathiny in chapter 8, Leon moved effortlessly between meaningful interactions with individuals and advocating for higher-level change. Three days before he died, he joined Mayor Lenny Curry and seven other healthcare leaders in the city for a news conference about the alarming rise in cases of coronavirus in the city — the previous week, one of every five new cases of COVID-19 in the United States was detected in Florida — and imploring residents to get vaccinated.[26] The Friday morning before his death, he was on a conference call with elected officials and community leaders in Jacksonville, continuing to urge increased attention to mitigation strategies and a greater focus on addressing vaccine hesitancy. And on Friday afternoon, before leaving for Palm Beach, he walked the floors of the hospital, encouraging his staff to get vaccinated and personally administering the dose to those who agreed.

Of all the health system leaders I've met, Leon stood out for his humility, curiosity, and respect for his workforce, as well as his willingness to explore unconventional approaches when those he served spoke up and told him the traditional ones were failing them. He was a remarkable man, gone too soon, but a model of transformative leadership for the future.

Conclusion

Nearly every time I give a talk or lead a seminar on moral injury, someone asks me to tell them how we can fix our broken healthcare system. Before exploring how to change things for the better, though, I usually begin by discussing the root cause of most moral injury. To get ourselves out of this mess, it's essential we understand how we got here.

The corporate drive for ever-increasing earnings and executive pay has transformed healthcare from a mission-driven industry into one motivated largely by revenue. The for-profit Health Management Associates got into hot water with the Department of Justice when CEO William Schoen chased profits by any means necessary, just as he had in the brewing business. But even nonprofit healthcare organizations have adopted the mantra "No margin, no mission."

American corporations weren't always so ruthless. When Matt Ramsey was a young boy in Schenectady, General Electric was still known as "Generous Electric." The company saw itself as a steward of its employees, its customers, and the communities where it operated, not just its shareholders.

Then came economist Milton Friedman. In his 1970 *New York Times* essay "A Friedman Doctrine: The Social Responsibility of Business Is to Increase its Profits," Friedman argued that a company is responsible only to its shareholders. The job of its chief executive is thus "to conduct the business in accordance with [shareholder] desires, which generally will be to make as much money as possible."[1] Individual shareholders could support social justice movements using their dividends, but the company need not concern itself with things like employee welfare or customer satisfaction, unless they threatened the bottom line. Therefore, Friedman concluded, "there is one and only one social responsibility of business — to use its resources and engage in activities designed to increase its profits."

The Friedman doctrine might have languished in the ivory tower if not for Jack Welch, who became the CEO of General Electric in 1981. Welch, argues David Gelles in his 2022 book, *The Man Who Broke Capitalism*, put Friedman's philosophy to work, "unleashing changes that transformed the company founded by Thomas Edison from an admired industrial behemoth known for quality engineering and laudable business practices into a sprawling multinational conglomerate that paid little regard to its employees and was addicted to short-term profits. And we all went along for the ride."[2]

During his twenty years as CEO, Welch turned GE into the most valuable company in the world. In his quest to enrich himself and his investors, Gelles says, Welch slashed his workforce; bought other companies, then broke them up and sold them for parts to turn a quick profit; and created a finance division that functioned as a giant unregulated bank. At one point, Welch hit his numbers for nearly eighty quarters in a row and everybody — shareholders and executives alike — wanted a piece of that pie. "An entire generation of managers sought to emulate his techniques, his growth strategies, and his values," Gelles concludes. "Welch redefined how corporations measure success, setting the standard for a generation of business titans." His thinking was codified by business school curricula and reshaped corporate legal theory.

Over the past forty years, a diaspora of former GE executives ascended the ranks of corporations around the country, such as Boeing, Albertson's grocery stores, snowmobile maker Polaris Industries, 3M, and Home Depot,[3] bringing his seemingly simple formula for success with them. CEOs like William Schoen introduced his hard-nosed strategies and creative accounting tactics to healthcare, consolidating an industry that was once made up mostly of small community hospitals and extracting enormous profits for themselves and their shareholders.

Though I had been talking for years about how the Friedman doctrine broke healthcare, I couldn't figure out why our society so readily accepted health systems more focused on profits than patient care. After reading *The Man Who Broke Capitalism*, it finally made sense. Jack Welch embodied the American Dream — a kid from a working-class family in small-town New England becoming one of Forbes 400 Richest Americans. As the first CEO widely revered by the general public, he built a massive following despite laying waste to towns like Schenectady, in part by declaring that what looked like greed was actually ethical behavior.

Men like my father, a small-time salesman, worshipped Welch even as he destroyed the GE plant in Pittsfield, Massachusetts, that made up a sizable chunk of his business. As Roger Martin, the former dean of the Rotman School of Management at the University of Toronto, put it to Gelles, the message was: "It may be sad that I've got to shut down this town, shut down this factory, but it's the moral thing to do." My father didn't understand how GE could post sky-high returns while he watched their factories crumble — no one did — but instead of looking for answers, he and his friends looked the other way, happy to take their fatter retirement funds at face value while imagining themselves the next Jack Welch.

But even if healthcare corporations and executives steeped in "Welchian" management demand fealty, as doctors our patients must come first. The bravest among us have already begun the fight to take medicine back. Doctors, with the support of a few administrators, blew the whistle on HMA, and clinicians like Ray Brovont from chapter 12 have led the charge to hold their employers responsible for patient safety.

At the heart of nearly every conversation we have had with clinicians in the last five years is some version of "this wasn't what I signed up for," a nagging sense that the covenant between physicians and their employers is broken. One day we will all be patients. Don't we want our health systems to put us, and the people who care for us, first?

Fortunately, resistance to shareholder primacy, and the devastation it reaps, may have already begun. The Business Roundtable, a group of CEOs from some of the largest corporations in the United States founded in 1972 by the influential leaders of General Electric, US Steel, and Alcoa, was originally created to support free market policies. In 1997, when Welch was at the pinnacle of his power, the group recommended the Friedman doctrine as the sole guiding principle for corporations. But the subprime mortgage crisis, which began in 2008, generated strenuous public outcry against corporate excesses; though the Occupy Wall Street protests lasted just fifty-nine days, the critique of capitalism reverberated in policy conversations for a decade.[4]

In 2019, the Roundtable openly disavowed shareholder primacy, declaring "the success of our system is dependent on inclusive long-term growth"[5] and returning to a much older definition of what a company was for and a commitment to a broader group of stakeholders — not just shareholders, but also employees, communities, and society.[6] The Roundtable even called out healthcare as one of the industries in need of new principles of corporate governance. The following year, the influential Davos Manifesto presented at the World Economic Forum in Switzerland echoed this sentiment.

With no hard evidence that business leaders have made any changes in light of the announcement, many analysts have dismissed it as little more than a publicity stunt to appease a more socially conscious, purpose-driven consumer base.[7] Nevertheless, the declaration exists and it is now up to us, whether we are shareholders, employees, or community members, to hold healthcare leaders to this guidance.

As more clinicians understand their distress as moral injury rather than individual frailty, they are increasingly willing to stand up to corporate recklessness. Since the first days of the pandemic when healthcare workers felt abandoned by organizations that failed to provide sufficient personal protective equipment, interest in unions has exploded. In January 2021, Mary Kay Henry, the president of the Service Employees International Union, told the *New York Times*, "In my 40 years of organizing health care workers, I have never experienced a time when people are more willing to take risks and join together to take collective action. That's a sea change."[8]

But what other specific steps can we take to build better healthcare systems? Over the past five years, many organizations have contacted us asking for help. As in the case of UF Health Jacksonville, they usually reached out after trying a range of programs to address rampant burnout in their workforce, but until one of their clinicians brought up how useful it was to reframe their distress as moral injury, they didn't understand why the problem persisted.

It would certainly be convenient if we could offer a turnkey program that relieved clinician distress, but there's no way to know which specific changes will be effective before doing the hard work of investigating the unique circumstances in each organization that cause problems. In general, though, we see less moral injury in organizations where doctors and other clinicians are full partners in organizational decision making, and leadership is open and responsive to clinician feedback. In such an environment, tracking systemic drivers of moral injury such as electronic medical record usage and tying executive compensation to measures of clinician well-being can be effective ways to make sure clinician distress remains a focus long-term.

The best way to show someone what change looks like is to point them toward organizations doing things better. After all, William Schoen learned to lead from stories about Jack Welch and his protégés. Some leaders of organizations in this book where physicians thrive are doctors, like Matt Ramsey and Jerry Williams in chapter 10, Mark Labuski and Joe Bellissimo in chapter 11, and Leon Haley from chapter 13, but many are not, like Ed Tufaro from chapter 10 and Leon's mentor, John Haupert, in chapter 13. What they have in common is an ironclad commitment to the mission of serving patients and a sense of responsibility to a broad group of stakeholders. They also model a way of leading with humility that everyone in healthcare can learn from.

First, they listen to their workforce. Leon Haley, from the previous chapter, spent time in clinical areas almost daily, and Mark Labuski, Joe Bellissimo, and Ray Brovont continued working as clinicians. Ed Tufaro, in chapter 10, does not have a clinical background, but he follows the advice of an early mentor to trade his suits for scrubs on a regular basis, and he actively looks for ways his operations team can better serve clinicians. There is simply no substitute for ground truth.

Strong organizations partner with clinicians to make decisions that affect patient care, such as establishing operating room teams or organizing workflow in a clinic. This can look like Rothman and Tristán, where the physician owners of the practice make decisions about operations; like the dyad model at Penn State, where physicians and administrators with equal say are paired at each level of leadership to help each other make the best decisions for their patients; or like Leon Haley's executive team, which was replete with physicians, including even positions more typically filled by business experts.

Finally, none of the physicians I profiled went into medicine for the money; the work is too hard and too heartbreaking for that. Administrators in this book, including non-clinicians like Ed Tufaro, are similarly mission-driven, putting patient care first even when it is hard to hold that line. The Tristán partners made financial sacrifices rather than accepting working conditions that would compromise their oath. Rita Gallardo, Jerry Williams, and Matt Ramsey walked away from stable jobs when they understood their employers did not share their commitment to putting patients first. And Ray Brovont spoke up, even when it cost him his job, and took on a multibillion-dollar corporation, in service to every future patient of his health system, and every future physician plaintiff, fighting to right corporate wrongs. No amount of money could make up for the distress these doctors would suffer if they were forced to betray their patients.

Sometimes even the most conscientious leaders, like Leon Haley and Mark Labuski, feel their hands are tied by red tape — policies, legislation, and regulations at local, state, and federal levels. Changing an industry that makes up one-sixth of the economy will require sweeping changes at every level of governance. Short of socializing the whole system, there are many concrete steps Congress could take at the federal level to rein in the detrimental fixation on profit margins in healthcare. What follows are just a few examples.

To start, Congress could put strict limits on consolidation and vertical integration by healthcare corporations, since there is no evidence it leads to either better outcomes or lower costs for patients. As we saw in chapters 6 and 11, the Federal Trade Commission has made some progress in this area, ruling against St. Luke's in their acquisition of Saltzer Medical Group in 2013 and against the proposed merger of Penn State Hershey and Pinnacle Health in 2014, but enforcement has been inconsistent and failed to prevent highly consolidated regions. When President Biden nominated Lina Khan to chair the Federal Trade Commission, she promised greater scrutiny of healthcare mergers. During her first two years, she has been true to her word. In February 2022, for example, she concurred with suing to block the merger of Rhode Island's two largest healthcare systems, Care New England and Lifespan, which owned Rhode Island Hospital when I worked there. In a letter describing the decision, she pledged continued vigilance not only about the consequences for patient care, but also about the implications of consolidation for the healthcare labor market.

Chairperson Khan's own words, in an address to a pharmacy group on June 22, 2022, best describes the power individuals have to effect change.

> There is nothing inevitable about the current structure of the market or the current business practices that occur and are permitted — these are all the result of policy and legal choices, that were made by public officials, and that can also be remade by public officials through the democratic process . . . The responsibility for crafting how our healthcare markets work is divided among dozens of state and federal authorities who are ultimately accountable to elected members of local, state, and federal legislative bodies . . . I hope everybody here — the patient advocates, the pharmacists, the other healthcare providers, and the concerned citizens — will remain fully engaged to ensure your voices are heard at all levels of government.[9]

In other words, at every level of government we must choose our elected officials carefully, and we must invest the time to educate them about our experiences, as clinicians and as patients. Those officials will decide whether healthcare corporations serve all their stakeholders, or continue to focus just on their shareholders.

Researching hospital executive backgrounds for this book, I found the trail goes cold after four or five years. It's very hard to find information about executive performance unless there were high-profile lawsuits or notable awards. Because executives are making decisions that impact patient care, it is time to hold them to standards consistent with those for physicians, whose infractions are cataloged in perpetuity in the National Practitioner Data Bank. If Congress established a Healthcare Executive Data Bank, health systems might think twice before hiring people like Mike Young and David Kreye, with track records of misconduct or mismanagement.

Regulation and legislation for the sake of patient safety are impossible to argue against. Yet the demands for documentation have gotten so unwieldly that meeting them can lead to inefficient and even inattentive care, and the consequent moral injury is driving people like

Mary Franco and Don Kovacs out of medicine altogether. Congress could demand that federal agencies further harmonize, consolidate, and reduce requirements for documentation and reporting to federal insurers, a task Seema Verma began tackling in 2017 when she became the administrator of the Centers for Medicare and Medicaid Services. By the time she left in 2021, Verma had reduced the overall number of measures in the CMS Medicare fee-for-service programs by 15 percent, from 534 to 460,[10] saving an estimated 3.3 million hours of reporting effort, as well as $128 million for the agency. The next administrator, Chiquita Brooks-LaSure, set the goals of fully electronic quality assessment and increased patient participation, and renamed the effort Meaningful Measures 2.0.[11] This work must continue and include clinician voices in future measures development.

Finally, Congress should take on insurance reform, because so much moral injury stems from the reimbursement process: Billing justifications require time-consuming notes that bloat the electronic medical record and do not improve care; prior authorization steals time from patients and delays necessary tests or treatment; a labyrinth of pharmacy formularies decided by kickbacks in closed-door deals between pharmaceutical companies and pharmacy benefit managers working on behalf of insurers makes it nearly impossible to prescribe the medication that's best for the patient's condition and for their wallet.

Ending prior authorization, a burden that amounted to $31 billion in lost clinician productivity in 2009, and which physicians say is getting worse every year, would be a huge step toward reducing clinician distress.[12] When I worked at Rhode Island Hospital, I spent more time chasing prior authorizations than I did face-to-face with patients. Prior authorizations aren't just time consuming, they also put lives at risk: One-quarter of physicians say that delays in care from prior authorization led to a patient's hospitalization.[13] Fed up with a wasteful practice with almost no demonstrable benefit, in 2021, Texas legislators passed a bill that gives doctors three years of immunity from prior authorization if 90 percent of their requests were approved during the previous six months.[14] That bill is a solid first step toward reducing moral injury, but we recommend taking the action further by making insurers prove a doctor is not following evidence-based medicine before requiring they submit prior authorizations.

Health insurance also must be easier for everyone to understand, so doctors like Blake Alkire don't face the moral injury of recommending treatments that unintentionally inflict financial harm. The Center for Consumer Information and Insurance Oversight, a division of CMS, was established by the Affordable Care Act of 2010 and charged with making health insurance more comprehensible for consumers, much as the Consumer Financial Protection Bureau did with the consumer credit industry in the wake of the economic crisis in 2008. Yet nearly a decade after the CCIIO was established, the Kaiser Family Foundation study cited in chapter 9 showed that 44 percent of employees still find their health insurance coverage, with numerous contingencies such as in-network status and the site of service delivery, impenetrable.

On July 1, 2022, an executive order signed by President Trump went into effect requiring insurers to disclose their negotiated rates for five hundred common procedures; by January 1, 2024, they must disclose rates for all procedures. Such transparency is laudable, but impossible for most individuals to parse. We recommend reforming the CCIIO to mirror the Consumer Financial Protection Bureau, enforcing usable transparency, educating patients about their insurance, and serving as a single place for complaints. If reform proves impossible, we urge Congress to start fresh by creating a new agency in that model.

Public policy changes, though imperative, are always slow to implement. Sometimes physicians ask us what they can do, right away, to make a difference. I always advise them to study the policy, regulatory, legislative, and financial constraints at play in the organizations where they work, much as Ray Brovont did when he laid the groundwork for his lawsuit against EmCare. Understanding the pressures under which their administrators operate will help them determine the most effective way to stand up and speak out about potential moral injury in their particular organization.

In July of my fourth year of medical school, I did an elective rotation on the trauma surgery service, thinking that might be my career. Thirty years later, two memories from that month still haunt me: the unique olfactory assault of the trauma bay — tequila, vomit, and the metallic tang of hemorrhage — and the deep uneasiness of the team when a young, fit patient rolled through the doors after a bad wreck, awake and talking even though their belly was full of blood.

Young patients have significant physiologic reserves, so their bodies can offset the damage of severe injuries for a long time. Yet only a rookie trusts how they "look," because when the last of their reserves are spent, all at once they crash. After sweating through one near miss, clinicians learn to anticipate the worst with these young patients, setting up resuscitation protocols and putting the blood bank and operating room on standby as soon as they get to the trauma bay.

Our work on moral injury for the past five years has reminded me of those patients. Like young trauma patients, physicians have deep reserves of resilience.[15] They can "look good" for a long time, despite experiencing extreme distress, until suddenly, they are not okay at all. For Matt Ramsey from chapters 1 and 10, that moment came when he witnessed his health system betray his mentor; for Jay Neufeld from chapter 6, it was the disregard for his patients' safety when his leadership failed to find someone to share call with him; for Rita Gallardo from chapter 7, it was when her employer sold the cancer clinic she had built without consulting her; for Blake Alkire from chapter 10, it was realizing that his care might cause his patients financial ruin; and for Ray Brovont from chapter 12, it was the death of a patient because the company he worked for refused to adequately staff his emergency room.

In the face of such betrayals, these doctors had to make a choice. They could throw up their hands and tell themselves that working in healthcare in the United States requires compromises. But if they succumbed to moral injury, they knew they were consenting to their own destruction. So they chose to fight — for their integrity as physicians, for their patients, and for the profession of medicine. May all of us be inspired by their courage. Together we can ensure that health systems enable physicians to practice as they were trained to do, putting patients first.

Notes

Introduction

1. Glenview Partners presentation to HMA board. July 2013. https://www.10xebitda.com/wp-content/uploads/2016/11/Glenview-HMA-Presentation-Jul-2013.pdf.

2. https://www.cnbc.com/2020/02/12/charlie-munger-warns-there-are-lots-of-troubles-coming-because-of-too-much-wretched-excess.html.

3. https://archive.knoxnews.com/business/union-leads-protest-at-hma-shareholders-meeting-ep-360815115-356995921.html.

4. https://www.americanprogress.org/article/rural-hospital-closures-reduce-access-emergency-care.

5. https://www.energy.gov/sites/prod/files/2013/11/f4/glass_vision.pdf; Alexander B. *The Glass House* (New York: Picador, 2017).

6. https://news.usc.edu/21941/Hospital-Chairman-Named-to-USC-Board.

7. https://www.nytimes.com/1974/02/09/archives/a-look-at-why-city-brewery-industry-went-flat-a-look-at-why-citys.html.

8. https://www.nytimes.com/1970/03/15/archives/long-private-schaefer-thrives-as-a-public-issue.html.

9. https://theschaeferstory.wordpress.com/chapter-iv.

10. https://brookstonbeerbulletin.com/historic-beer-birthday-rudolph-j-schaefer-iii; https://brookstonbeerbulletin.com/tag/schaefer.

11. http://jameskristie.blogspot.com/2009/07/bob-lear-something-he-never-forgot.html.

12. https://www.courant.com/hc-xpm-2011-09-18-hc-exlife-20110918-story.html.

13. https://www.washingtonpost.com/archive/business/1978/07/05/puerto-rico-enacts-tax-to-help-beer-industry/7753403a-fbf4-4cf9-a627-f5dcac597f10.

14. Moyer DG. *American Breweries of the Past* (Bloomington, IN: Author House, 2009).

15. Greene J. *Dare to Succeed: Experience the Satisfaction of Doing Business by the Book* (self-published, 2021).

16. https://championsofdestiny.com/business-leader-or-lunatic.

17. http://www.fundinguniverse.com/company-histories/health
    -management-associates-inc-history.

18. https://www.tampabay.com/archive/1999/06/14/a-prescription-for-profits.

19. https://www.tampabay.com/archive/1999/06/14/a-prescription-for-profits.

20. https://www.encyclopedia.com/books/politics-and-business-magazines/
    health-management-associates-inc.

21. https://www.theatlantic.com/health/archive/2015/04/the-problem-with
    -satisfied-patients/390684.

22. https://www.corporatecrimereporter.com/wp-content/uploads/2014/01/
    emcare.pdf.

23. https://www.pennlive.com/editorials/2011/08/adequate_nurse_staffing_
    levels.html.

24. https://www.justice.gov/opa/pr/hospital-chain-will-pay-over-260-million
    -resolve-false-billing-and-kickback-allegations-one.

25. https://www.beckershospitalreview.com/hospital-executive-moves/
    hma-confirms-new-board-of-directors.html.

26. https://www.healthcarefinancenews.com/blog/chs-hma-merger-creates
    -healthcare-behemoth.

27. *Schoen v. Health Mgmt. Assocs., Inc.* Case No: 2:14-cv-411-FtM-29CM
    (M.D. Fla. Aug. 25, 2015).

28. https://www.healthcarefinancenews.com/blog/chs-hma-merger-creates
    -healthcare-behemoth.

29. Hay Group. The Hay Group Study on Health Care Plan Design and
    Cost Trends, 1988 through 1997. National Association of Private Health
    Care Systems and National Alliance for the Mentally Ill, 1998. https://
    www.nabh.org/wp-content/uploads/2018/06/Health-Care-Plan-Design
    -and-Cost-Trends-REPORT-text-Black-White.pdf.

30. https://psychnews.psychiatryonline.org/doi/full/10.1176/pn.36.12.0017a.

31. https://cdn.mdedge.com/files/s3fs-public/Document/September
    -2017/0903CP_Malpractice.pdf

32. https://cdn1.sph.harvard.edu/wp-content/uploads/sites/21/2019/01/
    PhysicianBurnoutReport2018FINAL.pdf.

33. Patel RS et al. Factors Related to Physician Burnout and Its Consequenc-
    es: A Review. Behav Sci (Basel). 2018 Oct 25; 8(11): 98. DOI: 10.3390/
    bs8110098.

34. Kaschka WP, Korczak D, and Broich K. Burnout: a fashionable
    diagnosis. Dtsch Arztebl Int. 2011 Nov; 108(46): 781-87. DOI: 10.3238/
    arztebl.2011.0781. Epub 2011 Nov 18. PMID: 22163259; PMCID:
    PMC3230825.

35. National Academies of Sciences, Engineering, and Medicine; National Academy of Medicine; Committee on Systems Approaches to Improve Patient Care by Supporting Clinician Well-Being. *Taking Action Against Clinician Burnout: A Systems Approach to Professional Well-Being* (Washington, DC: National Academies Press, 2019 Oct 23). PMID: 31940160.
36. https://icds.uoregon.edu/wp-content/uploads/2015/03/Litz-et-al-2009 -Moral-Injury-and-Moral-Repair-in-War-Veterans.pdf.
37. Shay J. *Achilles in Vietnam* (New York: Simon & Schuster, 1995).
38. Morgan A, Shah K, Tran K, and Chino F. Racial, Ethnic, and Gender Representation in Leadership Positions at National Cancer Institute–Designated Cancer Centers. JAMA Netw Open. 2021 Jun 1; 4(6): e2112807. DOI: 10.1001/jamanetworkopen.2021.12807. PMID: 34097046; PMCID: PMC8185594; https://catalyst.nejm.org/doi/full/10.1056/CAT.21.0166.

Chapter 1

1. https://www.facs.org/-/media/files/archives/shg-poster/2016/14_halsted .ashx.

Chapter 2

1. https://www.cdc.gov/nchs/data/hus/2017/089.pdf.
2. https://www.ivantageindex.com/wp-content/uploads/2020/02/CCRH_ Vulnerability-Research_FiNAL-02.14.20.pdf.
3. Litvak E, and Bisognano M. More Patients, Less Payment: Increasing Hospital Efficiency in the Aftermath of Health Reform. Health Aff (Millwood). 2011 Jan; 30(1): 76–80. DOI: 10.1377/hlthaff.2010.1114. PMID: 21209441.
4. https://www.pennlive.com/news/2017/03/pinnaclehealths_planned_ acquis.html.
5. https://www.healthdesign.org/chd/research/culture-change-and-facility -design-model-joint-optimization.
6. https://www.regioner.dk/media/7613/the-use-of-single-patient-rooms-v -multiple.pdf.
7. https://www.jhconline.com/construction-under-bedded.html.
8. https://www.acpjournals.org/doi/10.7326/m16-0961.
9. Ofri D. The Business of Health Care Depends on the Exploitation of Doctors and Nurses. *New York Times.* 2019 Jun 8.
10. https://www.justice.gov/opa/pr/hospital-chain-will-pay-over-260-million -resolve-false-billing-and-kickback-allegations-one.

11. https://cumberlink.com/news/local/doj-hma-to-pay-260-million-to
-resolve-false-billing-allegations-carlisle-hma-pleads-guilty/article
_61ab6325-1f86-5cde-8865-e4019354d626.html.

12. https://fortune.com/fortune500/2013/community-health-systems-inc;
https://www.businesswire.com/news/home/20130730005773/en/Comm
unity-Health-Systems-to-Acquire-Health-Management-Associates.

13. https://vsg-law.com/wp-content/uploads/2016/08/US-ex-rel-Meyer
-Cowling-et-al-v-HMA-Newsome-EmCare-et-al-11-cv-1713-JFA
-Complaint.pdf.

14. Parsons D and Ray E. The United States Steel Consolidation: The
Creation of Market Control. J Law Econ. 1975; 18(1): 181–219. Retrieved
2021 Jul 19 from http://www.jstor.org/stable/725250.

15. https://www.hanys.org/communications/publications/healthcare_intelli
gence_reports/docs/2019-03_vertical_integration_report.pdf.

16. http://www.sfu.ca/~kawasaki/Elbaum.pdf.

17. https://www.upmc.com/about/why-upmc/story.

18. https://www.beckershospitalreview.com/largest-hospitals-and-health
-systems-in-america-2019.html.

19. https://www.massgeneralbrigham.org/who-we-are; https://www
.bostonglobe.com/2021/12/10/business/mass-general-brigham-reports
-profitable-year-despite-covid-challenges.

20. https://www.bostonglobe.com/2021/12/10/business/mass-general
-brigham-reports-profitable-year-despite-covid-challenges; Beckers
(https://www.beckershospitalreview.com/largest-hospitals-and-health
-systems-in-america-2019.html); https://fortune.com/company/
hca-holdings/fortune500.

21. https://issuu.com/herald-mail1/docs/fcmc_2020_anniversary_book.

22. https://fcmcpa.org/history.

23. https://www.healthexec.com/topics/covid-19/pausing-elective-operations
-cost-hospitals-22b-2020.

Chapter 3

1. Burman ME, Hart AM, Conley V, Brown J, Sherard P, and Clarke PN.
Reconceptualizing the Core of Nurse Practitioner Education and
Practice. J Am Acad Nurse Pract. 2009 Jan; 21(1): 11–17. DOI:
10.1111/j.1745-7599.2008.00365.x. PMID: 19125890.

2. https://www.brookings.edu/wp-content/uploads/2018/12/Steinwald_
Ginsburg_Brandt_Lee_Patel_GME-Funding_12.3.181.pdf.

3. Institute of Medicine (IOM). *Computer-Based Patient Record: An Essential Technology for Health Care* (Washington, DC: National Academies Press, 1991). DOI: 10.17226/18459.

4. https://www.commonwealthfund.org/publications/newsletter-article/federal-government-has-put-billions-promoting-electronic-health.

5. https://www.govinfo.gov/content/pkg/FR-2016-05-09/pdf/2016-10032.pdf.

6. https://archive.nytimes.com/www.nytimes.com/interactive/2012/09/25/business/25medicare-doc.html.

7. https://www.vox.com/2017/1/9/14211778/obama-electronic-medical-records.

8. https://khn.org/news/death-by-a-thousand-clicks.

9. Fuchs V. Major Trends in the US Healthcare Economy Since 1950. N Engl J Med. 2012; 366: 973–77. DOI: 10.1056/NEJMp1200478.

10. https://www.nextech.com/blog/healthcare-data-growth-an-exponential-problem.

11. https://khn.org/news/thousands-of-primary-care-practices-close-financial-stress-of-covid.

12. https://www.medscape.com/viewarticle/954066; https://www.ama-assn.org/about/research/employed-physicians-now-exceed-those-who-own-their-practices.

Chapter 4

1. https://www.statnews.com/2018/08/21/moral-injury-clinicians-healing.

2. https://www.justice.gov/archive/ndic/pubs40/40392/40392p.pdf.

3. https://about.kaiserpermanente.org/our-story/our-history/dr-sidney-garfield-on-medical-care-as-a-right.

4. Gerontology Institute, University of Massachusetts Boston. *The Older Population in Massachusetts, 1980–1990* (Gerontology Institute Publications, Paper 93, 1992).

5. https://books.google.com/books; Butler AM, Todd JV, Sahrmann JM, Lesko CR, and Brookhart MA. Informative Censoring by Health Plan Disenrollment Among Commercially Insured Adults. Pharmacoepidemiol Drug Saf. 2019; 28(5): 640–48. DOI: 10.1002/pds.4750.

6. https://www.govinfo.gov/content/pkg/GAOREPORTS-HEHS-94-119/html/GAOREPORTS-HEHS-94-119.htm.

7. https://books.google.com/books (p. 134–147).

8. https://commonwealthmagazine.org/opinion/my-take-on-mass-general
-brighams-financial-spin; https://www.massgeneralbrigham.org/.

9. https://catalyst.nejm.org/doi/full/10.1056/CAT.17.0558.

10. Freyd J, and Birrell P. *Blind to Betrayal: Why We Fool Ourselves We Aren't Being Fooled* (Chichester: Wiley, 2013).

11. Sinsky et al. COVID-Related Stress and Work Intentions in a Sample of US Health Care Workers. Mayo Clin Proc. 2021 Dec 1; 5(6): 1165–73.

Chapter 5

1. Ayvaci ER, Pollio DE, Hong BA, and North CS. Longitudinal Cost of Services in a Homeless Sample with Cocaine Use Disorder. J Soc Distress Homeless. 2019; 28(2): 132–38. DOI: 10.1080/10530789.2019.1598618; Fitzpatrick-Lewis D, Ganann R, Krishnaratne S, Ciliska D, Kouyoumdjian F, and Hwang SW. Effectiveness of Interventions to Improve the Health and Housing Status of Homeless People: A Rapid Systematic Review. BMC Public Health. 2011 Aug 10; 11: 638. DOI: 10.1186/1471-2458-11-638. PMID: 21831318; PMCID: PMC3171371; Wright BJ, Vartanian KB, Li H-F, Royal N, and Matson JK. Formerly Homeless People Had Lower Overall Health Care Expenditures After Moving into Supportive Housing. Health Aff. 2016; 35(1): 20–27.

2. https://www.hhs.gov/civil-rights/for-individuals/special-topics/community-living-and-olmstead/index.html.

3. https://nccppr.org/wp-content/uploads/2017/02/ncs_mental_health_system_where_we_have_been_where_we_are_and_where_we_are_headed.pdf.

4. Krebs A. Harry J. Anslinger Dies at 83; Hard-Hitting Foe of Narcotics. *New York Times.* 1975 Nov 18.

5. https://www.govinfo.gov/content/pkg/STATUTE-77/pdf/STATUTE-77-Pg282.pdf.

6. https://www.cms.gov/CCIIO/Programs-and-Initiatives/Other-Insurance-Protections/mhpaea_factsheet.

7. Barton WE. Trends in Community Mental Health Programs. Hosp Community Psychiatry. 1966 Sep;17(9):253–58. doi: 10.1176/ps.17.9.253. PMID: 5947932.

8. https://www.nami.org/NAMI/media/NAMI-Media/Infographics/NAMI_YouAreNotAlone_2020_FINAL.pdf.

9. Substance Abuse and Mental Health Services Administration. *Key Substance Use and Mental Health Indicators in the United States: Results*

from the 2016 National Survey on Drug Use and Health (HHS Publication No. SMA 17-5044, NSDUH Series H-52). (Rockville, MD: Center for Behavioral Health Statistics and Quality, Substance Abuse and Mental Health Services Administration, 2017). Retrieved from https://www .samhsa.gov/data.

10. Holly C, Andrilla A, et al. Geographic Variation in the Supply of Selected Behavioral Health Providers. Am J Prev Med. 2018;54(6):S199 –S207. Available at https://www.ajpmonline.org/article/S0749-3797(18)30005-9/fulltext.

Chapter 6

1. https://recordinglaw.com/united-states-recording-laws/one-party -consent-states/idaho-recording-laws.

2. https://www.medscape.com/viewarticle/940672.

3. Gorman A. For Doctors Who Take a Break from Practice, Coming Back Can Be Tough. KHN (Kaiser Health News). 2015 Jun 15. https://khn.org/ news/for-doctors-who-take-a-break-from-practice-coming-back-can -be-tough.

4. https://www.jointcommission.org/-/media/tjc/documents/resources/ patient-safety-topics/sentinel-event/sea_40.pdf.

5. https://www.psqh.com/julaug06/disruptive.html.

6. Rosenstein AH, O'Daniel M. Disruptive Behavior and Clinical Outcomes: Perceptions of Nurses and Physicians. Am J Nurs. 2005 Jan;105(1):54–64; quiz 64–65. doi: 10.1097/00000446-200501000-00025. PMID: 15659998.

7. Hall LH, Johnson J, Watt I, Tsipa A, O'Connor DB. Healthcare Staff Wellbeing, Burnout, and Patient Safety: A Systematic Review. PloS One. 2016;11:e0159015.

8. Shanafelt TD, Balch CM, Bechamps G, Russell T, Dyrbye L, Satele D, Collicott P, Novotny PJ, Sloan J, Freischlag J. Burnout and Medical Errors Among American Surgeons. Ann Surg. 2010 Jun;251(6):995–1000. doi: 10.1097/SLA.0b013e3181bfdab3; Brown SD, Goske MJ, Johnson CM. Beyond Substance Abuse: Stress, Burnout, and Depression as Causes of Physician Impairment and Disruptive Behavior. J Am Coll Radiol. 2009 Jul;6(7):479–85. doi: 10.1016/j.jacr.2008.11.029. PMID: 19560063.

9. https://www.nytimes.com/2019/06/08/opinion/sunday/hospitals -doctors-nurses-burnout.html.

Chapter 7

1. https://fas.org/sgp/crs/natsec/RS22452.pdf.
2. https://www.army.mil/article/173808/survival_rates_improving_for_soldiers_wounded_in_combat_says_army_surgeon_general.
3. https://www.army.mil/values.
4. https://ssl.armywarcollege.edu/dclm/pubs/study1970.pdf.
5. https://warroom.armywarcollege.edu/special-series/anniversaries/my-lai-a-stain-on-the-army.
6. https://press.armywarcollege.edu/cgi/viewcontent.cgi?article=1996&context=parameters.
7. https://www.healthcarestrategy.com/wp-content/uploads/2016/02/Ellsworth-Tarr-Wayne-Boydell_Misc_2014.pdf.
8. https://fibroblast.com/wp-content/uploads/2018/10/Patient-Leakage-A-new-survey-highlights-high-costs-limited-control-October-2018-1.pdf.
9. Barnett ML, Song Z, Landon BE. Trends in Physician Referrals in the United States, 1999–2009. Arch Intern Med. 2012;172(2):163–70. doi: 10.1001/archinternmed.2011.722.
10. https://www.admere.com/amr-blog/four-ways-healthcare-providers-can-reduce-referral-leakage.
11. Brot-Goldberg Z, de Vaan M. Intermediation and Vertical Integration in the Market for Surgeons. Unpublished manuscript, University of California, Berkeley, 2018.
12. Venkatesh S. The Impact of Hospital Acquisition on Physician Referrals. Unpublished manuscript, Carnegie Mellon University, Pittsburgh, PA, 2019. https://shruthi-venkatesh.github.io/publication/working-paper-2.
13. https://marketware.com/leakage-splitter-behavior/?gclid=CjwKCAjwsNiIBhBdEiwAJK4khsYDHzh2vb--_0Owcmo96Ba248TP2CKYvWRzB3t2GITfmawWwfvJPhoCjB8QAvD_BwE.
14. https://www.admere.com/amr-blog/four-ways-healthcare-providers-can-reduce-referral-leakage.
15. Koch T, Wendling B, Wilson NE. Physician Market Structure, Patient Outcomes, and Spending: An Examination of Medicare Beneficiaries. Health Serv Res. 2018;53(5):3549–68.
16. Scott KW, Orav EJ, Cutler DM, Jha AK. Changes in Hospital Physician Affiliations in US Hospitals. Ann Int Med. 2018;168(2):156–57.
17. https://fibroblast.com/wp-content/uploads/2018/10/Patient-Leakage-A-new-survey-highlights-high-costs-limited-control-October-2018-1.pdf.

Chapter 8

1. https://www.inquirer.com/business/health/tower-health-closing-brandy wine-jennersville-hospital-20211209.html.

2. https://www.philaworks.org/wp-content/uploads/2020/10/Philaworks -Quarterly-LMI-Report-April-2021.pdf.

3. https://www.thelancet.com/action/showPdf?pii=S0140-6736%2802% 2911824-1.

4. https://www.youtube.com/watch?v=4n1hQOeZOoM.

5. https://www.youtube.com/watch?v=4n1hQOeZOoM.

6. inquirer.com/philly/opinion/commentary/opioids-emergency-doctor -wolf-disaster-declaration-20180112.html.

7. https://www.governor.pa.gov/newsroom/governor-wolf-declares-heroin -and-opioid-epidemic-a-statewide-disaster-emergency.

8. https://www.govinfo.gov/content/pkg/USCOURTS-paed-2_20-cv -00127/pdf/USCOURTS-paed-2_20-cv-00127-0.pdf.

9. https://armandalegshow.com/wp-content/uploads/2022/06/Web -Transcript-S7-Ep04_Docs-vs-PE-.pdf.

10. https://www.inquirer.com/opinion/commentary/jennersville-rural -hospital-pennsylvania-chester-closed-20220127.html.

11. https://www.inquirer.com/opinion/commentary/jennersville-rural -hospital-pennsylvania-chester-closed-20220127.html.

12. https://books.google.com/books?id=0yOp5Ci5_EEC&pg=RA2-PA3&lp g=RA2-PA3&dq=hill+burton+funds+jennersville+hospital&source= bl&ots=M6GUMV8zhA&sig=ACfU3Uo8aHH5SyMMoARnQh6x KLThud-RGw&hl=en&sa=X&ved=2ahUKEwiB97WS-PD2AhUkNX oKHdToBwAQ6AF6BAgbEAM#v=onepage&q=hill%20burton%20 funds%20jennersville%20hospital&f=false (page 255).

13. https://www.bizjournals.com/philadelphia/stories/2001/07/16/daily11 .html.

14. https://www.bizjournals.com/philadelphia/stories/2001/07/16/daily11 .html.

15. https://www.healthcaredive.com/news/chs-community-health-systems -q4-full-year-2017-earnings/517986.

16. businesswire.com/news/home/20170929005734/en/Dommunity -Health-Systems-Completes-Diverstiture-of-Five-Pennsylvania-Hospitals.

17. https://www.inquirer.com/business/health/tower-health-plans-hospitals -sale-bids-drexel-mckinsey-20210428.html.

18. https://towerhealth.org/articles/reading-health-system-completes -acquisition-five-hospitals-region.

19. https://www.inquirer.com/business/health/tower-health-plans-hospitals
    -sale-bids-drexel-mckinsey-20210428.html.

20. https://www.inquirer.com/business/health/tower-health-hospital-layoffs
    -covid-19-20200616.html.

21. https://towerhealth.org/articles/tower-health-announces-actions
    -strengthen-system-ensure-long-term-mission.

22. https://www.documentcloud.org/documents/21087732-tower-chester
    -county-tax-decision?responsive=1&title=1.

23. http://canyonatlantic.com.

24. https://www.inquirer.com/business/health/tower-health-brandywine
    -jennersville-hospital-closure-lawsuit-20220128.html.

25. https://archive.naplesnews.com/news/local/new-east-naples-hospital
    -ceo-is-well-traveled-ep-401055212-344360492.html.

26. https://insurancenewsnet.com/oarticle/Government-records-depict
    -money-troubles-at-Lakeway-hospital-%5BAustin-American-St-a-404532;
    https://www.healthcarefinancenews.com/news/university-general
    -health-system-files-bankruptcy-after-failed-acquisition#:~:text=The%20
    Houston%2Dbased%20University%20General,put%20its%20finances
    %20in%20peril.

27. https://www.bizjournals.com/philadelphia/news/2021/12/09/tower
    -health-canyon-brandywine-jennersville-deal.html.

Chapter 9

1. https://www.kff.org/report-section/the-burden-of-medical-debt
    -introduction.

2. https://www.census.gov/library/stories/2021/04/who-had-medical-debt
    -in-united-states.html.

3. Himmelstein DU, Lawless RM, Thorne D, Foohey P, and Woolhandler
    S. Medical Bankruptcy: Still Common Despite the Affordable Care Act.
    Am J Public Health. 2019; 109: 431–33. DOI: 10.2105/AJPH.2018.304901.

4. https://www.cnbc.com/2019/06/25/medical-debt-not-student-loans
    -could-force-you-into-bankruptcy.html.

5. https://www.nature.com/articles/s41572-022-00341-1.

6. https://www.nytimes.com/2019/02/21/well/live/the-financial-toxicity
    -of-illness.html.

7. https://files.kff.org/attachment/Report-KFF-LA-Times-Survey-of-Adults
    -with-Employer-Sponsored-Health-Insurance.

8. Shrime MG, Weinstein MC, Hammitt JK, Cohen JL, and Salomon JA.
    Trading Bankruptcy for Health: A Discrete-Choice Experiment. Value

Health. 2018 Jan; 21(1): 95–104. DOI: 10.1016/j.jval.2017.07.006. Epub 2017 Sep 1. PMID: 29304947; PMCID: PMC6739632.

9. Alkire B, Hughes CD, Nash K, Vincent JR, and Meara JG. Potential Economic Benefit of Cleft Lip and Palate Repair in Sub-Saharan Africa. World J Surg. 2011 Jun; 35(6): 1194–201. DOI: 10.1007/s00268-011-1055-1. PMID: 21431442.

10. Abbott MM, Alkire BC, and Meara JG. The Value Proposition: Using a Cost Improvement Map to Improve Value for Patients with Nonsyndromic, Isolated Cleft Palate. Plast Reconstr Surg. 2011 Apr; 127(4): 1650–58. DOI: 10.1097/PRS.0b013e318208d25e. PMID: 21460672.

11. https://www.lancetglobalsurgery.org/_files/ugd/346076_713dd3f8bb5947 39810d84c1928ef61a.pdf.

12. https://www.nytimes.com/2021/08/22/upshot/health-care-prices-lookup .html.

13. https://www.cancernetwork.com/view/financial-toxicity-part-ii-how-can -we-help-burden-treatment-related-costs.

14. Baicker K and Chandra A. Medicare Spending, the Physician Workforce, and Beneficiaries' Quality of Care. Health Aff. 2004; 23: w184–97. DOI: 10.1377/hlthaff.w4.184. Published online 2004 Apr 7.

15. https://www.medscape.com/slideshow/2019-malpractice-report-6012303 ?src=ban_malpractice2019_desk_mscpmrk_hp#1.

16. https://www.ama-assn.org/sites/ama-assn.org/files/corp/media-browser/ public/government/advocacy/policy-research-perspective-medical-liability -claim-frequency.pdf.

17. https://www.healthsystemtracker.org/chart-collection/health-spending-u -s-compare-countries-2/.

18. https://www.commonwealthfund.org/publications/fund-reports/2021/ aug/mirror-mirror-2021-reflecting-poorly.

19. https://www.nytimes.com/2009/03/05/us/politics/05obama-text.html.

20. https://www.newyorker.com/magazine/2009/06/01/the-cost-conundrum.

21. Institute of Medicine (IOM). *Value in Health Care: Accounting for Cost, Quality, Safety, Outcomes, and Innovation* (workshop summary). (Washington, DC: National Academies Press, 2010).

22. IOM. *Best Care at Lower Cost: The Path to Continuously Learning Health Care in America* (Washington, DC: National Academies Press, 2013).

23. Shrime MG, Weinstein MC, Hammitt JK, Cohen JL, and Salomon JA. Trading Bankruptcy for Health: A Discrete-Choice Experiment. Value Health. 2018 Jan; 21(1): 95–104. DOI: 10.1016/j.jval.2017.07.006. Epub 2017 Sep 1. PMID: 29304947; PMCID: PMC6739632.

Chapter 10

1. https://hbr.org/2013/12/the-hidden-benefits-of-keeping-teams-intact.
2. Huckman R. The Hidden Benefits of Keeping Teams Intact. Harv Bus Rev. 2013 Dec.
3. Muhly W. Sustained improvement in intraoperative efficiency following implementation of a dedicated surgical team for pediatric spine fusion surgery. Perioper Care Oper Room Manag. 2017 Jun; 7: 12–17.
4. Hang Cheng et al. Prolonged Operative Duration Is Associated with Complications: A Systematic Review and Meta-Analysis. J Surg Res. 2018 Sep; 229: 134–44. DOI: 10.1016/j.jss.2018.03.022; Childers CP, Maggard-Gibbons M. Understanding Costs of Care in the Operating Room. JAMA Surg. 2018; 153(4): e176233. DOI: 10.1001/jamasurg.2017.6233.
5. Reznick D, Niazov L, Holizna E, Keebler A, and Siperstein A. Dedicated Teams to Improve Operative Room Efficiency. Perioper Care Oper Room Manag. 2016; 3: 1–5.
6. https://www.uphs.upenn.edu/paharc/features/creation.html.
7. https://www.athenahealth.com/knowledge-hub/practice-management/expert-forum-rise-and-rise-healthcare-administrator.
8. https://www.jec.senate.gov/public/index.cfm/republicans/2010/8/america-s-new-health-care-system-revealed.
9. Hamel Z. The End of Bureaucracy. Harv Bus Rev. 2018 Nov–Dec.
10. https://cmglaw.com/articles/which-defendants-do-you-name-in-a-medical-negligence-case.
11. https://www.doholis-lambert.com/blog/responsibility-without-authority-dysfunctional-delegation.
12. https://www.nytimes.com/1995/12/13/us/university-agrees-to-pay-in-settlement-on-medicare.html.
13. https://www.thedp.com/article/2006/01/back_from_the_brink.
14. Courtney PM, Darrith B, Bohl DD, Frisch NB, and Della Valle CJ. Reconsidering the Affordable Care Act's Restrictions on Physician-Owned Hospitals, J Bone and Joint Surg. 2017 Nov 15; 99(22): 1888–94. DOI: 10.2106/JBJS.17.00203.
15. https://goodjobsinstitute.org/what-is-the-good-jobs-strategy.

Chapter 11

1. https://www.pennlive.com/midstate/2011/03/remembering_theodore_tristn_of.html.

2. https://www.nytimes.com/2007/06/19/health/19docs.html.
3. Levin DC and Rao VM. The Effect of Self-Referral on Utilization of Advanced Diagnostic Imaging. Am J Roentgenol. 2011; 196(4): 848–52.
4. https://www.ahra.org/AM/Downloads/OnlineEd/2006NovemberDecember2.pdf.
5. US Government Accountability Office, Letter to Senators John D. Rockefeller IV and Gordon H. Smith Regarding Medicare: Trends in Fees, Utilization, and Expenditures for Imaging Services Before and After Implementation of the Deficit Reduction Act of 2005. 2008 Sep 26. https://www.gao.gov/assets/100/95803.pdf.
6. https://www.modernhealthcare.com/article/20161017/NEWS/161019923/penn-state-pinnacle-drop-merger-after-appeals-court-loss.
7. https://www.beckershospitalreview.com/hospital-physician-relationships/radiology-hospitals-biggest-opportunity-needs-a-quality-standard.html.

Chapter 12

1. https://www.beckershospitalreview.com/legal-regulatory-issues/missouri-physician-collects-26m-in-wrongful-termination-lawsuit.html.
2. https://mississippitoday.org/2020/04/05/two-mississippi-doctors-fired-after-speaking-out-about-coronavirus-safety; https://www.npr.org/sections/health-shots/2020/05/29/865042307/an-er-doctor-lost-his-job-after-criticizing-his-hospital-on-covid-19-now-hes-sui.
3. Plantz SH, Kreplick LW, Panacek EA, Meht T, and McNamara RM. A National Survey of Board-Certified Emergency Physicians: Quality of Care and Practice Structure Issues. Am J Emerg Med. 1998; 16: 1–4; McNamara RM, Beier K, Blumstein H, Weiss LD, and Wood J. A Survey of Emergency Physicians Regarding Due Process, Financial Pressures, and the Ability to Advocate for Patients. J Emerg Med. 2013 Jul; 45(1): 111–16.e3. DOI: 10.1016/j.jemermed.2012.12.019. Epub 2013 Apr 18. PMID: 23602793.
4. https://www.medpagetoday.com/infectiousdisease/covid19/85869.
5. https://www.tampabay.com/news/health/doctor-says-she-was-fired-for-reporting-low-staffing-at-brandon-regional/2218497; Heilman JA, Tanski M, Burns B, Lin A, Ma J. Decreasing Time to Pain Relief for Emergency Department Patients with Extremity Fractures. BMJ Qual Improv Rep. 2016; 5(1): u209522.w7251. DOI: 10.1136/bmjquality.u209522.w7251.
6. https://www.npsfoundation.org/trustees/leonard-riggs; https://www.zippia.com/envision-healthcare-careers-3986/history.

7. https://www.modernhealthcare.com/article/19940801/NEWS/408010325/healthcare-services-ipos-in-first-half-of-1994-chart.

8. https://sec.report/Document/0000950152-03-005679.

9. AMA Advocacy Resource Center. Issue Brief: Corporate Practice of Medicine. 2015

10. https://www.nytimes.com/1997/07/31/business/laidlaw-agrees-to-buy-emcare-for-336-million.html.

11. https://www.courant.com/news/connecticut/hc-xpm-1999-09-14-9909140156-story.html.

12. https://www.chieftain.com/story/special/1999/09/17/laidlaw-plans-to-sell-local/8783259007.

13. https://www.trailer-bodybuilders.com/archive/article/21728164/laidlaw-in-bankruptcy.

14. https://www.latimes.com/archives/la-xpm-2003-jun-24-fi-rup24.8-story.html.

15. https://www.onex.com/about/overview.

16. https://www.nber.org/system/files/working_papers/w29874/w29874.pdf.

17. https://www.onex.com/static-files/34ee3ef8-8d32-4468-939a-4a8a5b6 0abb3; https://www.forbes.com/sites/elliekincaid/2018/05/15/envision-healthcare-infiltrated-americas-ers-now-its-facing-a-backlash/?sh=13e 37a4e284f.

18. https://www.nytimes.com/2017/07/24/upshot/the-company-behind-many-surprise-emergency-room-bills.html.

19. https://www.cdr-inc.com/news/press-release/clayton-dubilier-rice-completes-3.2-billion-acquisition-emergency-medical.

20. https://www.cbc.ca/news/business/onex-sells-u-s-medical-investment-1.1102276.

21. https://www.sec.gov/Archives/edgar/data/1578318/000104746915001498/a2223319z10-k.htm.

22. https://www.aaem.org/UserFiles/MarApr16Editor.pdf.

23. https://hcavsamerica.org/wp-content/uploads/2022/02/SEIU_Investigative_Report_FINAL-1.pdf.

24. https://www.courts.mo.gov/file.jsp?id=167435.

25. https://u.pcloud.link/publink/show?code=BOl.

26. https://www.courts.mo.gov/file.jsp?id=167435.

27. https://u.pcloud.link/publink/show?code=BOl.

28. https://www.courts.mo.gov/file.jsp?id=167435.

Chapter 13

1. https://mediasite.video.ufl.edu/Mediasite/Play/577f8b51de5a47d0ad2be
   d0ee81c68131d.
2. https://www.nytimes.com/1990/07/29/magazine/the-tragedy-of-detroit
   .html.
3. Lewin ME and Altman S, editors. *America's Health Care Safety Net: Intact
   but Endangered Institute of Medicine Committee on the Changing Market,
   Managed Care, and the Future Viability of Safety Net Providers* (Washington, DC: National Academies Press, 2000).
4. https://mediasite.video.ufl.edu/Mediasite/Play/577f8b51de5a47d0ad2be
   d0ee81c68131d.
5. Ragin DF, Hwang U, Cydulka RK, Holson D, Haley LL Jr, Richards CF,
   Becker BM, and Richardson LD. Emergency Medicine Patients' Access
   to Healthcare (EMPATH) Study Investigators. Reasons for Using the
   Emergency Department: Results of the EMPATH Study. Acad Emerg
   Med. 2005 Dec; 12(12): 1158–66. DOI: 10.1197/j.aem.2005.06.030. Epub
   2005 Nov 10. PMID: 16282515.
6. https://smhs.gwu.edu/urgentmatters/sites/urgentmatters/files/CareMan
   agementUnitImprovesEDFlow.Grady__0.pdf.
7. Kohn LT, Corrigan JM, and Donaldson MS, editors. *To Err Is Human:
   Building a Safer Health System* (Washington, DC: National Academy
   Press, Institute of Medicine, 1999).
8. https://smhs.gwu.edu/urgentmatters/sites/urgentmatters/files/confer
   ence_materials_2004_Agenda_Sessions_2004.pdf.
9. https://www.ajc.com/news/local/grady-ceo-apologizes-for-shine-shoes
   -remark/OS9lbtvxvDqHzAvD8oH7gP.
10. https://www.georgiahealthnews.com/2017/02/notoriously-tough-job
    -grady-chief-survives-thrives.
11. https://www.healthleadersmedia.com/strategy/qa-grady-memorial-hospi
    tals-new-ceo-john-haupert.
12. King M. *A Spirit of Charity: Restoring the Bond Between America and Its
    Public Hospitals* (Salisbury, MD: Secant Publishing, 2016).
13. https://www.georgiahealthnews.com/2017/02/notoriously-tough-job
    -grady-chief-survives-thrives.
14. https://mediasite.video.ufl.edu/Mediasite/Play/577f8b51de5a47d0ad2be
    d0ee81c68131d.
15. https://ufhealthjax.org/about/documents/economic-contributions-2018
    .pdf.

16. https://www.visitjacksonville.com/about/jax-facts.

17. https://www.census.gov/quickfacts/jacksonvillecityflorida.

18. https://ufhealth.org/sites/default/files/media/PDF/139742_1.6.20-UFH_ Community_Benefit_Report_FY19_Fnocrops.pdf.

19. https://www.firstcoastnews.com/article/news/health/uf-health-facing-95 -million-challenge/77-123498557.

20. https://med.jax.ufl.edu/news/story/?id=2874.

21. https://ufhealthjax.org/about/mission-vision-and-values.aspx.

22. https://smhs.gwu.edu/urgentmatters/sites/urgentmatters/files/CareMan agementUnitImprovesEDFlow.Grady__0.pdf.

23. https://www.dvidshub.net/news/338004/hospital-corpsmen-graduate -trauma-training-program-naval-hospital-jacksonville.

24. https://news.wjct.org/first-coast/2018-07-23/mayor-pitches-120-million -for-uf-health-jacksonville-as-hospital-braces-for-other-cuts.

25. https://www.bizjournals.com/jacksonville/news/2021/10/21/dr-leon-haley -community-impact-award.html.

26. https://brooksrehab.org/news/mayor-curry-hospital-administrators -provide-covid-19-update.

Conclusion

1. Friedman M. A Friedman Doctrine — The Social Responsibility of Business Is to Increase Its Profits. *New York Times*. 1970 Sep 13.

2. Gelles D. *The Man Who Broke Capitalism: How Jack Welch Gutted the Heartland and Crushed the Soul of Corporate America — and How to Undo His Legacy* (New York: Simon and Schuster, 2022).

3. https://www.investmentnews.com/former-ge-executives-successful-as -ceos-elsewhere-5070.

4. https://time.com/6117696/occupy-wall-street-10-years-later.

5. https://s3.amazonaws.com/brt.org/archive/legacy/uploads/studies-reports /downloads/BRT_History_11720II.pdf; https://opportunity.business roundtable.org/ourcommitment.

6. https://perma.cc/3NAK-SCDQ.

7. https://www.forbes.com/sites/bobeccles/2020/08/19/an-open-letter-to -the-business-roundtable-181/?sh=3e57eb064001; Bebchuk LA and Tallarita R. Will Corporations Deliver Value to All Stakeholders? Vand L Rev. 2022; 75(4). Available at https://ssrn.com/abstract=3899421. DOI: 10.2139/ssrn.3899421; Raghunandan A and Rajgopal S. Do Socially Responsible Firms Walk the Talk? 2021 Apr 21. Available at https://ssrn .com/abstract=3609056. DOI: 10.2139/ssrn.3609056.

8. https://www.nytimes.com/2021/01/28/health/covid-health-workers -unions.html.

9. https://www.ftc.gov/system/files/ftc_gov/pdf/Remarks-Lina-Khan -Economic-Liberties-National-Community-Pharmacists-Association.pdf.

10. https://www.cms.gov/files/document/2021-cms-quality-conference-cms -quality-measurement-action-plan-march-2021.pdf.

11. https://www.cms.gov/newsroom/press-releases/speech-remarks-cms -administrator-seema-verma-2020-cms-quality-conference.

12. Casalino LP, Nicholson S, Gans DN, Hammons T, Morra D, Karrison T, and Levinson W. What Does It Cost Physician Practices to Interact with Health Insurance Plans? Health Aff. 2009; 28(Suppl 1): w533–43; https:// www.ama-assn.org/system/files/prior-authorization-reform-progress -update.pdf.

13. https://www.ama-assn.org/system/files/prior-authorization-survey.pdf.

14. https://legiscan.com/TX/bill/HB3459/2021.

15. West CP, Dyrbye LN, Sinsky C, et al. Resilience and Burnout Among Physicians and the General US Working Population. JAMA Netw Open. 2020; 3(7): e209385. DOI: 10.1001/jamanetworkopen.2020.9385.

Acknowledgments

While writing this book, the willingness of so many to share so much with me, simply for the hope that it could make a difference, repeatedly surprised me. There would be no book but for those who are named or anonymized here, who provided background facts and corroboration, or whose stories may not appear, yet enriched these chapters. Not all of those I spoke with were physicians; lawyers, veterinarians, educators, physical therapists, pharmacists, social workers, and others trusted me with their struggles of moral injury, too. Both for those I've named and for those I cannot — who know who they are — I am humbled by, and indebted to, your courage.

It is a rare opportunity to work with someone who is so perfectly complementary that your mutual effort only moves forward, in huge leaps. There is no better thought partner than Simon Talbot, who is psychologically astute, intellectually curious, brave, clear, unassuming, generous, impish, and whose processing speed is almost unmatched. It has been an honor to work together for the past eight years, pushing boundaries and accountability wherever we see the need. May we continue for many more years to come.

Physicians might still be struggling for accurate language for their distress had Pat Skerrett at STAT News not been bold enough to publish our first article. The entire moral injury movement is indebted to him, as are we.

Stephen Bergman, a.k.a. Samuel Shem (author of *The House of God*), believed the world needed this book and, over dinner at his house in May 2019, convinced us it was possible. His persistence and guidance got Simon and me past early hurdles, which were mostly our own doubts.

Our luckiest break was finding a publisher with vision, willing to take a huge risk. Chip Fleischer grasped the concept of moral injury during our first conversation. He trusted an untested team to bring an amorphous concept into a fully evolved "big idea" that could speak truth to power and offered the resources and time we needed to make it better than we dreamed. What a rare thing, indeed.

Chip's most brilliant gift was to suggest developmental editor Rebecca Radding. Working with a new writer who is unfamiliar with the emotional, intellectual, and structural landscape of writing creative nonfiction is not for the faint of heart. Rebecca's patience, persistence, compassion, honest assessments ("huh?"), and humor made what could have been agony into an intensive but rewarding "writing residency." I will forever hear her incisive editing voice as I write. Thank you for taking the journey with me, Rebecca.

My family takes after Parvin, generous in every way, and I am thankful every day for those echoes of her. Shervin, Austin, and Caleb bore with me, without complaint, through the years of experiences that shaped this book — frustration, career changes, extensive travel, long stints when I worked nonstop without a paycheck — and the months of actual writing, when simple things like having food in the house, much less on the table, was a gamble, if left to me. Those three men are, simply, what makes my world go 'round and every reason I work for better.

Thanks, for various reasons — reading countless drafts; wrangling schedules; offering a meal, a distraction, or a brief respite; bearing emotional burden when the book's content was raw; pushing me to think harder; offloading animal care so I could focus; or helping me wrestle business concepts to the ground — to Megan Lloyd Thompson, Tom Thompson, Elizabeth Holman, Konrad Weatherhogg, Grace D'Alou, Mary and Ed Franco, Deborah Morris, Keith Corl, Ira

Bedzow, Moshe Cohen, Elena Perea, Jim Beckner, MacKenze Burkhart, John and Allison Getz, Janet and Richard Holman, Lisa Suzenski, Marissa Smith, Ariel Morton, Lambros Georgallas, each of the 1,500 members of Physician Women Equestrians, Felicitas von Neumann-Cosel, Larisa Rose, Izzy Beaumont, Carlos, Eva, Darby, Chad Zeaser, and Kyle Milne.

And finally, my gratitude to two wise mentors who have fundamentally changed how I think: Don Berwick, whose early conversations reassured us we were on the right track; and Charles ("Hutch") Hutchinson, who saw my potential decades before I did and never wavered in his conviction.

Dr. Wendy Dean left clinical medicine when generating revenue crowded out the patient-centered priorities of her practice. Her focus since has been on finding innovative ways to make medicine better for both patients and physicians through technology, ethics, and systems change.

Dr. Dean practiced for 15 years as an emergency room physician and then as a psychiatrist. After leaving clinical practice, she spent eight years in leadership positions, overseeing medical research funding for the US Army, and as a senior executive at a large nonprofit in Washington, DC, supporting novel strategies to restore form, function, and appearance to ill and injured service members. She turned her full attention to addressing moral injury in 2019.

Dr. Dean is a regular contributor to Medscape's "Business of Medicine"; blogs on *Psychology Today*; and continues to work in innovative fields with NASA, the American Society of Reconstructive Transplantation, and the Transplant Ethics and Policy Working Group at New York University Langone Medical Center.

Dr. Simon G. Talbot is a hand surgeon and microsurgeon who is Associate Professor of Surgery at Harvard Medical School and Attending Surgeon in the Division of Plastic Surgery at Brigham and Women's Hospital in Boston, Massachusetts.

Dr. Talbot's research focuses on nerve repair and the psychosocial aspects of hand and arm amputation and transplantation.

He graduated from the University of Auckland, School of Medicine in New Zealand. He completed his residency in the Harvard Plastic Surgery Residency Program followed by a fellowship in hand and microsurgery at Beth Israel Deaconess Medical Center.